Margaret Frings Keyes, author of *Inward
Journey*, has written extensively on crises in
the life cycle. A social-activist psychotherapist
with a private practice in San Francisco and
Muir Beach, California, she has developed a
form of intensive therapy, a 10-day residential
"incubation" period during which an individual works with a current crisis in terms of the
themes of his or her life and family-legacy
questions. Many of the art exercises, techniques for dream amplification, and journal
suggestions in *Inward Journey* have been
adapted from her methods of therapy.

The
creative
activity
of
imagination
frees
man
from
his
bondage
to
the
"nothing but"
and
raises
him
to
the
status
of
one
who
plays.
As
Schiller
says,
man
is
completely
human
only
when
he
is
at
play.

—C. G. Jung

THE REALITY OF THE PSYCHE SERIES

INWARD JOURNEY

Margaret Frings Keyes

JOURNEY

Art as Therapy

With New Supplement
on Active Imagination
by Marie-Louise von Franz

Photographs by Michelle Vignes
Cover art by Ivis Nasir

OPEN COURT
La Salle & London

responsibility that entails. The creative arts are one of the best ways to touch and experience this center and to promote healing.

The other dimension in self-understanding and self-healing (which is what I understand psychotherapy to be) is to use the materials of art in meditations with specific goals of understanding. Use of nonverbal means of expression, even for one unfamiliar with the full range of possibilities in an art medium, i.e., the naïve beginner without any skill, can allow one to connect with and express things that are understood in one's body—ideas and feelings that have been coded within us in forms without words. The use of a medium in which one is *not* skilled allows a slowing down to reconsider the "obvious," and often one finds it is not so obvious or there is more that wants to be known. This approach to self-knowledge is basic to the exercises outlined in *Inward Journey*. Again, however, the individual is the one interpreting his or her own experience, making his or her own exploration.

Some therapists have objected that the material elicited in such exercises is so deep that the methods should be restricted to the therapeutic setting where there are safeguards. On the contrary, I believe that when the question is ready to be asked, a guide can be found. For some it will be in the form of psychotherapy. Particularly in combining art with psychodrama, intense emotional affect can be released as the protagonist deals with his or her projections via the use of group members who represent the significant others in his or her life. The therapist contains and focuses this energy in a way that the individual working alone cannot.

The psychotherapist, however, is not the only guide. Many persons find their path to be a spiritual discipline; others find it in closely attending to the ordinary encounters of life. Individuals have been making the journey inward for at least as long as recorded history. It is my hope that this book will be useful for some on the path.

Two further notes on this edition. First, both men and women are referred to when the masculine gender is used. I regret that it was not feasible to revise the entire text to correspond to the greater consciousness of sexist language developed since the book was originally published. And, second, this edition includes a supplemental discussion of active imagination.

I wish to acknowledge the immeasurable debt I owe to those who have shared their journeys with me and given me permission to use their artwork and descriptive comments. Anita De Vall, Billie Kelly, and Janice Toby in particular gave invaluable assistance. Claire Philpott helped me to shape the original material. Joseph Wheelwright, M.D., his wife, Jane Wheelwright, and Mary Goulding, M.S.W., gave me criticism and encouragement. I express appreciation to Marie-Louise von Franz for the use of her supplement on active imagination. Finally, I am most indebted to Fritz Perls and Eric Berne, with whom I studied and whose theory has shaped so much of my practice.

MARGARET FRINGS KEYES

SAN FRANCISCO, CALIFORNIA
DECEMBER 1982

Introduction

ART AND PSYCHOTHERAPY

Men have always used the arts of music, poetry, dance, drama, painting, writing, and sculpture to symbolize, explore, and say what could not be said in words. The creative genius of other men's works illuminates the individual's situation, mirrors and deepens his questions. As a therapist, I can select and relate creative works to my client's condition to the degree I know the rewards in these forms—art can open directions for him to pursue. My concern here is to describe in practical detail how I use art materials with the nonartist, the client who has come into therapy with some very specific questions and problems. Some of these questions are similar to your own for they are the questions of anyone who seeks to understand himself, his thoughts, his feelings and actions.

These art processes, originally developed in work with troubled clients, I have used in workshops with teachers, students, ministers, and a range of people who simply wished to know themselves more deeply and who found these methods useful. This book is written for you to share these means and utilize them for your own self-growth.

A crisis is usually the precipitating agent to psychotherapy. Paradoxically, it is the unwanted divorce, the loss of a goal, the recognition of incapacity or inner emptiness, boredom or restlessness which opens the way to new growth by finally forcing a symbolic clearing of ground and pruning of dead forms. Men who have found that competition and achievement only lead to more of the same with diminishing flavor, women whose roles are changing before their eyes and who can no longer feel settled down in marriage and motherhood—realistically, the first step for them is to look at where they are.

In the treatment situation, this is done either individually or in a small group of people about the same age but with varying life circumstances. Although I work individually in a number of different ways, when the situation allows I prefer to start with a week of intensive treatment in which the client comes every day and works for whatever period of time something meaningful is happening.

This is a time of clearing away old self-images like unfinished business from the past with parents or spouse. It is a time of identifying recurring patterns of behavior and looking at the underlying questions they have been attempting to answer. And, it is a time of looking at how an individual now perceives himself—the changing body image, varying energy levels, specific talents, interests that may have been laid aside, training that may or may not be worth bringing up-to-date in terms of the person he now feels himself to be.

This first week characteristically releases a significant increase of energy and subjective feeling of well-being and self-value. Undoubtedly this is partially due to the repressed parts

I drew a picture of my fear. It seems to be a vortex with hands reaching out to pull me in.

being listened to and taken seriously, but also because the process itself brings an upwelling of forgotten memories, and the sense of self grows fuller as the roots and connections are seen.

There is no set way to begin treatment. In my practice, I often use videotape, initially setting the camera for a full body view and letting the client tell his story without interruption or comment. When he has finished we replay the tape and reset the camera for a close-up of his face as we discuss what he has seen. This too is replayed and allows the client to experience direct body data for the first time: the expressive use of his eyes and mouth, his style of interaction, his aggressiveness or hesitancy, his need to explain, or sometimes his lack of hearing, the areas of tension in his body and voice. Most people program their behavior and communication in terms of how they expect to be perceived. They modify behavior in terms of interactional cues, e.g., I see you wince when my voice is too loud, I tone down my voice and become more aware of my own excitement because I see your reaction.

The client, via the videotape, has access to direct information about himself that is not ordinarily available to him. This awareness itself causes a process of change. For example, Addie had remarkable physical beauty but a tight, querulous voice and an expression that went with it. They clearly did not fit her body. As we viewed the tape, she said she sounded and looked like her mother—her mother was very uncertain of her own value and place with her husband, a woman who had her daughter's teeth capped and nose bobbed, constantly talked to Addie about how fat she was, and who also gave and withheld gifts from her.

The therapy questions now became "Why was Addie still carrying her parent in her body?" and "What did this have to do with her difficulty?" She had periods of being unproductive in her profession during which she would gain huge amounts of weight. Such obvious and vivid feedback revealed an image of the parent which had been taken inside and it felt like Addie herself. This does not happen often but the client always sees some aspect of his behavior in a different light.

Art therapy does not answer the questions. It provides a process to clarify and deepen the questions, an awareness of how the individual here and now participates in creating his life conditions, and it points to some options that might be chosen. There are no highly visible models for this task. It is an individual journey. The individual has to take back parts of himself which he dislikes and does not want to see. He has to differentiate his own path from the ways of unthinking conformity to *what is done by most people.* He has to discover his own dark and negative side and the elements in his personality that are like those of the opposite sex. In order to make this discovery a family sculpture, a journal of dreams, beginning dialogue work, and Gestalt psychodrama will carry the process forward.

Art materials vivify the process and reach different levels of the personality than can words alone. Clay is used for its sensory, tactile qualities and capacity to bring out the as yet unworded. I particularly like to use it when I have someone who stays away from his feelings by analyzing and speculating on the *whys* of his behavior. In one instance I brought in a married couple for a completely nonverbal session. A partition was placed between them and each worked with clay to depict what their relationship felt like, then the relation to the most problematic parent for each, and finally to their child. At this session, looking at her husband's sculpture of a wall separating her from him and their son, the wife recognized how deeply her husband identified with their mentally defective son who had been placed in foster care immediately after infancy. The mother felt his care was too burdensome to her own career, and her husband felt he too was expendable to her driving ambition! As they talked she began to understand how much her ambition was a cover for her own feelings of vulnerability which were rooted in a reaction to the *helplessness* of her mother.

Clay is useful in the exploration of sticky, messy, bad feelings. Bob, a young doctor, used clay to smear and skin-print portions of his journal as he described and almost embodied his self-disgust, his anger, and his confusion about his need for love and approval which prevented him from showing other people either his anger or his strength. His treatment was complex as was his use of art materials. He used music and movement to express different kinds of feelings warring within him. Some of it was terrifying. He created two foam rubber sculptures—Good Mother and Bad Mother—one, soft and lovely, the other with wild eyes, a jagged mouth, and bloody vagina. At one point he jumped up, bit off her nipples, ripped a knife from his pocket and plunged it repeatedly into her body until he collapsed crying and sobbing with his arms around Good Mother. This session marked a turning point in treatment and in his relationship to me. He had previously been unable to express negative feelings towards his own mother or towards me. We were now able to talk about them and he had a series of psychodrama confrontations with his mother going back to different ages, telling her what he resented and how he was hurting. With role reversal (in which he acted and expressed the thoughts and feelings of his mother) he was able to reach some differentiation of his fantasies from what her reality may have been. With the inner dialogues (written conversations with characters from his dreams) and psychodrama exercises, he came to recognize the positive and negative female aspects in his own personality and the expressive needs these represented.

Inner dialogues are written when the client recognizes a dream character or element which behaves in a significant way in one or more dreams. He addresses several questions to the character and imagines the other's responses, in effect writing a dialogue much as in a play. This is useful; he gets in touch with knowledge he has but did not recognize. In psychodrama, the client describes a scene to me, either an actual past event (when Bob was eight years old, his father brought him a surprise, a horse; Bob was terrified and his father, angry and disgusted, called him a girl) or an anticipated encounter (Bob was planning to apply for a bank loan and anticipated feeling vulnerable and defensive). We imagine the stage and set it with what props are necessary in chairs and space and the client and I act it out. He plays each part and I change places with him becoming whatever other person is needed. We then act alternative ways of doing the same scene, sometimes just giving voice to the feelings and thoughts which had previously been unspoken. His understanding and control deepens as he recognizes emotionally more aspects of each situation, options for his future choices, and ways of saying goodbye and finishing situations with which he was burdened in the past.

Example of work with fiction to deepen understanding of aspects of self: *I have just read Charles Williams' novel DESCENT INTO HELL. This represents the two central characters—one man committed suicide yet found redemption through love. The other man climbs down a rope into hell with a self-centered love that becomes monstrous. They represent possible choices I see but have not looked at before.*

Psychotherapy to be effective has to provide a means for knowing and understanding both the world we have built and our activity in creating this world. Getting in touch with the mythic quality of life through literature and drama can help us to see the patterns we create in our own lives, particularly how our inner explanations of the way things are partially determine the outer events that happen to us.

Cassie, an ex-nun, provides an example of how this works. When I first met with her she did little but weep. The sessions contained long, blank pauses which seemed to accurately reflect the life she was leading. Living alone and working at a bookkeeping job that in no way reflected her intellectual ability or academic achievements, she took no initiative in establishing a social life and turned aside any attempts by others to get to know her. She described herself in the past as a victim of circumstances and the bad will of others. However, my perception of her strengths grew, particularly as she made good use of symbolism in fantasies. Her inward journey is more fully described later but here I wish to note how large amounts of related reading, much of it fiction, and one film facilitated her treatment.

She was not in touch with her own actions which maneuvered others into doing the *wrong thing* which she then judged as their fault and used to justify her victim role and immobility. I suggested she read Laurens van der Post's *Venture to the Interior*, a tale of an African safari that can also be read as a journey to the interior of the psyche, and two of Joseph Conrad's novels, *Heart of Darkness* and the *Secret Sharer*. She became more aware of her suppression of the dark side of her character, the anger and bad will which she had not owned and experienced as coming from others. She was much like the white men the books dealt with, who denied and feared their own instinctual nature. They scapegoated and projected their aggression and sexuality onto the natives. We used other books, Sheila Moon's *Knee Deep in Thunder*, a fantasy that describes a journey with some very strange characters and how they all are needed to manage various obstacles along the way. She came to identify various sub-personalities in herself, some of which she did not like, who nevertheless had an importance in managing her life. She went to the movie "Walkabout" (a story of an Australian aborigine who rescues and travels with a young woman and her brother; finally, not being really understood or seen, he dies). She recognized her situation in these art forms, saw that she had the option of responding and saying *yes* to newly discovered instinctual elements within her or *no* and letting them die. She did not let them die. She astonished me in a group session a couple of months later by casually remarking to one of the men, "You really turn me on." He did. They have been comfortably married for a couple of years now.

Art therapy is a life-quickening process. It is not meant to substitute for the relationships of the real world, but it provides means for comprehending them and for trying new behavior. The feeling of being fully alive and confident of their own ability to continue growth is at a peak when clients end the intensive phase of treatment. This tapers off in the months that follow, but in my follow-up one to two years later they generally report feeling more integrated than before and they know more about the stimuli to old patterns which they either avoid or use differently. There are lapses but also periods of remembering to remember that tide them over. More importantly, they have made decisions and tried out different behavior and they are being seen and related to by the people who matter to them in ways which confirm the direction they are going.

This book utilizes my experience as a psychotherapist, it is a guide for people undertaking this pilgrimage to knowing themselves. I will accompany you for a portion of the way, describing the journey inward with art experiences which will uncover (or discover) the ways in which you limit yourself, will show you the autonomy and choice you possess, and ways of awakening images from the inner depths to guide you in choosing direction. Then we will discuss the creative process as the central part of the inward journey in light of the three major systems of theory: Transactional Analysis, Gestalt Experience, and Jungian Depth Psychology.

Right now I am not in touch with the growing places or love from other people. I feel trapped in a well but I know I am not only the trapped part but that which can call out. I keep myself trapped by not calling out.

The Inward Journey   I.

DIRECTION

You are about to begin creating images that can guide you into your deeper self. In the course of your journey, art experiments are suggested which can evoke associations and insights into the wider dimensions within, underneath your conscious self. You must supply a space to work in, either a quiet room or a comfortable natural setting, and the materials. You can work alone or in a group.

A word about materials. Different aspects of you, like different personalities, need different art media to express what wants to be said. Since you will be acting out with materials and words the most neglected parts of yourself, you may need to experiment with a range of materials to find what feels right to express these feelings.

Some possibilities:

CLAY Slippery, gritty, oozy between your fingers, hardening, lumpy, good to pound, to carve when it is soft, to scratch when it is hard, to throw, fling, roll, pinch, shape, and create something that never existed before.

PAINT Large jars of poster paint that you can use to drip, dribble, and splash, maybe having run water over the drawing sheet beforehand to let the colors merge and blend and swirl out as you shake the page; explore brush possibilities (or sponge or twigs or your own fingers and hands) making all kinds of lines, wiggly, thin, wide, nervous, firm, strong, teasing with short strokes or long, looping, free, funny. You don't have to please anybody or make anything pretty, or neat, or significant.

CRAYONS AND OTHER COLOR Craypas are half crayons and half pastels—take the paper off so you can use the side for broad strokes, felt-tip pens, charcoal sticks, india ink—all have their own particular language possibilities. Wax crayons, rubbed hard on paper, resist colored inks painted over them and become brilliant, jewel-like lines or blotches.

Things can be combined. After paint has dried, a twig dipped into black india ink creates exciting line possibilities—try some with your awkward hand, the one you usually do not use in writing; it is freer to do things differently, not perfectly.

PAPERS AND COLLAGE MATERIALS Collage materials can be added with glue to papers of all kinds, newspapers, grocery sacks, slick surfaces, absorbent tissues. Collage materials can be almost anything but it is easy to start with portions of pictures cut from magazines, whatever catches your eye. Include old photographs of you, combine them to make some-

thing absurd, or to make a statement through connections that really interest you.

PLAY and DISCOVER!

In order to guide yourself, you must know where you are
before you begin the journey. And since you will be both the
explorer and the explored, you had best check your present
position and orient yourself clearly before you move from the
familiar you into areas that may seem strange and foreign. So,
to find out where you are now we will take the first step.

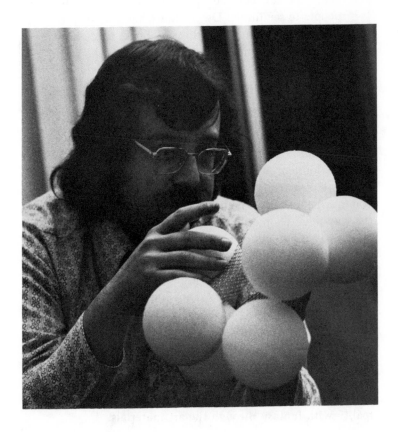

THE SELF BOX

Materials you will need: a cardboard box, scissors, glue, and a pile of old picture magazines. You are going to make a three-dimensional representation of you. It does not have to be a box, any shape with an inside and an outside will do.

Make something that feels right to you in terms of size, depth, breadth. Starting with a cardboard box, you can cut the openings that allow other people to see inside. Determine what you keep on the inside of you. What do you choose to show on the outside? Represent these. Paint if you choose or glue on parts of magazine pictures, materials, and favorite objects.

When you have finished, think about what you have placed in the center, what you have included that you prefer to keep hidden, what you have not included. If you are making this along with a group that will talk together after, you may be startled to realize you left out some major aspect of the way other people see you. Did you include anything from your past, any hopes or fears, what you feel bad about yourself, what you like about yourself? Add them now, if you wish.

How did you go about the process of constructing your image? Did you do it quickly, knowing with sureness the way it should be? Perhaps a bit carelessly, thinking more of the idea you wanted to represent rather than whether the construction would stand? Or did you feel your way slowly?

In making the Self Box you experienced yourself in an active, unique and unrepeatable way. You formed a visible, graphic record of your perception of you; you integrated your reality with fantasy through the art materials.

Oddly enough, everything you did shouted what you are. This construction is as uniquely you as your thumbprint or your handwriting. Your style in both the material you selected and the way you went about your construction, your process, can be seen as the essence of you shining through every choice.

"But I'm not an artist," you may protest, "if I were, this would look better." Skill with the use of art materials is not the point. You played with material and created possibilities with what you found. You are not concerned here with ART but with using materials to extend your awareness of your own experience possibilities. You want to rediscover the naive wisdom you had as a child. Of course you are not Picasso. You are you. You are finding out more about you and not comparing or ranking with anyone. You are *unique*.

Jennie, who most often thought of herself as a wife and mother, constructed a box made of mirrors on the outside. It was difficult to find the opening, but once inside the mirrors completely fell away and the box revealed pictures of deep sea creatures of intense color and beauty as well as pictures of dark painful wounds. As she talked of her box it became clear that she had spent her life reflecting what she thought the people around her wanted to see. She kept the dark side of life, her hurts and anger, hidden even from herself much of the time. The cost was high. Her vivid inner beauty was not visible either.

Ben, on the other hand, had a construction which seemed carelessly put together at first glance, yet on closer inspection, it held a wealth of detail. Images of masculine competitiveness vied for room with delicate flower-like women and sensuous fantasies. He had placed a small box within the larger one and this opened to a mathematically precise construction of wooden toothpicks. He was at a loss to account for this but somehow he knew it was important. There was something more in him to be discovered which he did not yet understand.

Two examples of self boxes: The top one covered with foil opens up to a world of color and organic forms. The lower box is meant to hang; it has passageways filled with a candle, feathers, wheat stalks, etc. A sea shell in the center is suspended in a net. Each represents how the maker felt about his inner life.

Your box may not be as elaborate as these but when it is finished, it too can tell you more than you knew you intended. Look at it carefully and notice the questions it raises. These are small signals of what needs to be explored and of what needs to be transformed on the journey you are beginning.

YOUR LIFETIME

Materials you will need: A large piece of paper at least 24" x 36", poster paints, felt-tip pens, or charcoal.

Imagine that this paper represents the whole of your lifetime, the beginning, the now, the future and the end. First sit quietly for a few minutes, then fill it however you choose. Don't expect anything, or try, or analyze, just allow your mind to be quiet, to let happen what will by simply holding the thought: *This is my lifetime.*

When you have finished be aware of the quality of your breathing and how your body feels, and how it felt to be totally absorbed with the making. Where do you feel the most excitement? What did you discover? What do you want to share?

Ann started clockwise from the lower part of her sheet with dull monochromatic colors for the portion which represented her childhood, gradually brightening them as she proceeded into young womanhood after the sad, dark, heavy lines representing her experience of high school, blazing out with joyful colors with the birth of her first child, shifting into clear blues and greens as she represented the struggle to define herself as a person loving and related to her family but separate from them. Three quarters around she left the future blank.

Molly approached the project from a completely different angle. In the top left corner of her sheet was a multicolored ball which gradually appeared to unravel across the page developing various angles and color possibilities. The whole sheet was covered with paint. "I haven't finished," she explained "but this is what I intend, to experience every possibility I can imagine."

Kate's picture looked more like a conventional landscape yet the symbols held specific meaning for her. A road, her life, stretched from the bottom left hand side of the page and seemed to disappear in the middle, a place of centering where a sun, conscious awareness, was rising. She placed a crescent moon, which to her represented the phases of her womanhood, over the sun. On the left, a tree with its forking roots visible stood by a stream, representing her inner experience with herself, and a mountain with a house on the right represented her relationship with others.

The three pictures, very different from one another, emerged as each woman faced the blankness of the sheet and allowed herself to feel what was the meaning of her lifetime and how to depict it. Each discovered a central theme or pattern. Two stressed how they *felt* about their lives; one, how she *thought* about it. Look at your lifetime painting. Does it show more about the way you think or about the way you feel about your life? Does it have a center or is it linear like an ongoing story? What are the themes and questions in it?

If you answer these questions with certainty, you are ready to move to the beginnings, how it all began, how you came to be you.

THE FAMILY SCULPTURE

Where your journey began and what baggage you have carried from that time.

When you were a child you got a lot of messages and instructions about how to be you from your family. You not only learned manners, how to dress, what friends to choose and such, but also you picked up some of your parents' attitudes towards life, particularly their view of your worth and your importance or lack of it. One way of exploring what these messages were is by sculpting what your family felt like when you were growing up.

What we are investigating in this chapter is how YOU came to think about yourself in the ways you do and perhaps limit yourself in the ways you do. You want to clear away distortions picked up from how other people have viewed you and how you have responded in order to reach the sense of you now deciding your own fate, setting your own goals.

THE FAMILY SCULPTURE

Materials you will need: a good double handful of clay, paper, and pencil.

First, close your eyes and go back to a time in your childhood, somewhere between two and eight years old. Think about the members in your family. Who was around? How old were they? How did you feel about them?

Note on the paper two or three adjectives describing each person. Take the clay and make a sculpture of the adjectives describing one particular person, e.g., if you described Dad as *warm but critical*, you might make just an arm reaching out

from a ball with a lot of sharp points. The idea is
not to make a figure of a person, but something that
gives a feeling of how that person felt to you when
you were younger.

When you have sculpted each family member
in turn, put them in relation to each other to show
who felt close and who was far away from you
emotionally. You might show who was on top and
who was under someone else in the family.

You now have a sculpture that shows what it
felt like to be growing up in the family into which
you were born. Look at it carefully and sense what
your sculpture might indicate that you had not
thought of before. Write one question or comment
from each family member in the sculpture to you,
and then your comment or question to each family
member.

The Family of Your Past

The way you discover how you got to be the way you are is to
look at the messages from the family of your birth and the
decisions you made about them. The messages you wrote from
the sculpture are some of the instructions you received about
what you should do and what to avoid to gain approval. You
may have been told how to be a winner; you may have been
told how to be a loser. Some of the problematic messages had
to do with *not* being you: "Be perfect"; "Don't be silly";
"Don't be a child."

As a child you learned to behave in ways that got you
some attention. Even if it was not the kind you wanted most, it
was better than none. Certain feelings or actions were associated with that attention: getting on the honor roll or playing
dumb, throwing a tantrum, being awkward and spilling

things, becoming a rebel, or being a victim to get comfort and feel justified—any one of these could have become a favorite role for manipulating the attention you needed.

Mother—*warm but engulfing*

Father—*mild mannered and unknown*

Sister—*awkward but interesting*

Jeremy—*affectionate and intelligent*

So much more comes out in the sculpture than can be said in words. Jeremy, a bright young lawyer, in doing his family sculpture pictured his mother *warm but engulfing* as a large mushroom in the center of the family circle, his father *mild mannered and unknown* a small lumpish object hidden from his view by the mother figure, and his sister *awkward but interesting* a squarish object with a large number of arm-like protuberances. He depicted himself as an ocean wave, a slightly less bulky figure than his mother but tending towards her form.

The central importance of his mother was clear, as was the absence of a direct relationship with his father and the similar structure of his own identity to that of his mother. Her messages to him were: "Don't be you. Be important as I would like to be." Jeremy had bought her program: he was active in school politics, president of his student body, head of his class in law school. Only now at 35 was he waking up to realize that he hated all forms of competition and that the profession for which he had prepared himself held no interest for him.

A good clue in understanding your own functioning is to think about the feeling with which you are most familiar now—competitive, jealous, angry, depressed, dumb. It just might be that you are collecting feelings of a particular kind. A feeling prompts you to use your energy to get your needs met, then the feeling goes away. If you have a particular feeling much of the time or in many situations, then chances are that you are not using it to identify what you want changed and doing something about it. Instead you are expecting someone else to do something and you are collecting that old familiar feeling that you used to associate with some kind of attention in your family. If showing hurt feelings in your family did not pay because they were ignored, you may have learned to attack with a temper tantrum which got some action. Today you might find when you are ready to explode with anger, you are actually hiding a feeling of hurt inside. The attention you got then and get now will never satisfy the hurt because it is not acknowledged. In Transactional Analysis this is known as a *Racket*. That is a rough word to use, but when you know that almost everybody has a favorite bad feeling he/she tends to collect, there is a bracing quality, almost like a cold shower, in calling your particular bad feeling a racket. This is especially true if it is something like feeling very unappreciated and sorry for yourself, or smoldering anger. It very quickly changes your accustomed way of looking at things. For example, you can begin to think about what kind of payoff you get from collecting such an ostensibly unhappy feeling. Do you cash it in for something else?

Jeremy discovered he was playing a blaming game of "If it weren't for you..." and "Now see what you've made me do." Staying immobilized and *confused* used to demonstrate to his mother that her ideas weren't so great. It did the same to other people who tried to direct or advise him now.

ANNA'S
FAMILY
SCULPTURE

Father—*distant, hardworking, knows
a lot*

Mother—*warm, angry, hurt*

Brother—*wanting love,
demanding
attention*

Anna—*bright, lonely, artistic*

Messages:

from father: "I don't want you. Work hard but you won't be successful."

from mother: "Be what I wanted to be (a dancer) but don't be sexy."

from brother: "Pay attention to me."

from Anna to parents: "I'll work hard at being what you want but I won't succeed and I won't be sexy."

to brother: "I'll pay attention to you rather than me."

When Anna depicted her family she realized she had received messages from her father that life was a struggle; she should work hard but since she was only a girl, she would not count for much. From her mother, Anna heard "Don't be sexy," but also that she should be someone special, probably a professional dancer as her mother had wanted to be. For a long time Anna took lessons, practiced and struggled to become a dancer. It did not occur to her that she had combined and was acting out her parents' directions—a struggling, nonsexy dancer was certainly not going to count for much!

A Racket feeling always covers up another feeling that could be used to change the situation, but for some reason that feeling was really scary to feel as a child, so the child used and started collecting this substitute feeling instead. In Anna's family, anger was quite unacceptable. Being sad on the other hand was O.K. and she could get a backrub or some attention. So gradually whenever there was stress or trouble and some anger would be called up in Anna, she learned to suppress it and feel sad instead. As time went on this felt quite natural, almost like that was how one should feel, e.g., helpless and sad when a bully took a toy instead of angry and capable of getting it back. As a result, Anna lost much of her power to take care of herself, which closely fitted her father's idea of what a woman was and confirmed his message that she *wouldn't count for much.*

Let's look again at your own family sculpture. Look at it for the feelings it sets up in you, then go over the list of messages from family members to determine the instructions which told you how to be, how to get attention, how to manage your life. Now look at your own messages to find out how you did or did not buy the program, the decisions you made about you. Children do not have to buy the destructive messages. But most of them do, a little. Jeremy had bought the "Don't be you, be what I want you to be." He now had to decide to be himself. Fortunately, most children grow up with two parents and often a grandparent or an older brother or sister who give them options in ways of looking at themselves.

Your Here and Now Family

We now have arrived at the second level of analysis—here and now. Look at each message again. Is anyone currently saying the same thing to you? Your boyfriend, girlfriend, boss, husband, wife, an associate? (It is almost incredible how many people find all, or nearly all, of the early messages now being sensed coming from their spouses.) To whom are you currently sending your old messages? If you discover there is a strong carry-over, you are now in a position to clear away some of the major distortions in your relationships. Anna was dismayed to realize she was sending the same messages she had received as a child now to her husband, i.e., "I don't know whether I want you; work hard but you won't be successful; pay attention to me."

The basic idea is that from your early decisions and feelings you probably built up a repertoire of two to five predictable sets of interactions with other people which you use to get the attention you feel you need. The setups you may be using to collect the familiar feelings can be infuriating to other people or fascinating and sometimes even amusing but they always serve to structure time and your energy in ways that prevent much real closeness to anyone and stifle growth.

It is important to understand the family messages or injunctions about how to be and your childhood decisions, in order to learn that you can make a new decision. This means a redecision on some of those crucial early injunctions you originally accepted. Anna, in the here and now of looking at her family sculpture, thought about where she was now hearing messages similar to those early ones. Although she had a tendency to think her husband did not value her sexually, she basically knew this message was coming from herself alone and she had never taken the risk of trying to be definitely attractive. She did not want to make mistakes which she thought would bring ridicule. When she probed this sore place she remembered feeling humiliated when she thought her father had laughed at her as a little girl in her first bathing suit. She now saw that keeping this memory was perhaps part of her early decision to collect sadness and follow mother's message not to be sexy. She realized that she never visited the boutique stores whose clothes intrigued her but instead shopped sales for sensible clothes. She looked at her well-tailored but drab dress of brown checks and added, "I hate this outfit. I feel like a stick in it. It's about time I made a redecision. I don't have to keep telling myself to buy clothes that will last and avoid the things that would be fun for only a single season."

Anna had moved to another level of looking at the family sculpture as a picture of herself, a depiction of aspects of the early family that she had hidden inside. In the language of psychology these are *introjects*. The introjected messages sound like they are coming from you. (When you hear the family messages coming from others, it is known as *projection*.) Introjected parent messages have a lot of *shoulds* and *oughts*. They are often phrased in the second person as you talk to yourself inside. Often they are variants, of course, of the messages you wrote from family members in your sculpture.

Anna, when she thought of the sculpture as a picture of herself, had to question what in her was like her strong masculine father? She determined this was her nursing role which she had developed after giving up the idea of a dancing career. She decided that a change was necessary in the sculpture as a picture of herself; the hurt feminine aspect of her needed to be cared for and helped to risk growing and the bright and curious child aspect in her needed more room to explore. She moved the clay figures closer.

"I choose to be me, not mother's idea of me, and that means connecting more with my body (here she placed the

sculpture of herself, a head with spikey bumps, on top of the
headless body of her infant brother sculpture). I love to dance
though not professionally. I love to make things and use my
hands. I haven't done this for years, but I choose to *now*. The
strong masculine and the wounded feminine aspects in me
make a good pair when they are related (here she placed the
masculine tower within the crescent of the feminine). I block
myself when I keep them apart."

Anna's work illustrates the meditative possibilities in working. As she looked at the problematic aspects of her family sculpture she began to sense the strengths and where certain feeling energy in the family had been misdirected. This raised questions, e.g., if her parents could have been more caring to one another, then could the parts of her which were like those parents, her masculine power and feminine vulnerability be brought closer? Her potential for becoming an integrated whole person became clearer. You might write a similar outline for your own sculpture.

Redecisions and Revisions

As some of the above works for you, come back to the sculpture again, looking at it now in terms of your goal of reaching a more creative, inclusive sense of self. You can't reject, deny, or throw out any part of what you have been, but you can work with it and come to a different relationship particularly with those parts you do not like and want to repress. You can find out what strengths there might be, what odd, perverse blessings these unchosen, unwanted aspects and experiences can hold for you. Often, just playing with the figures, putting them into different combinations, relating mother to father in a different way, can suggest possibilities about the interplay of your own strengths and weaknesses. Writing these insights, sharing them with another or others helps to strengthen the redecision. It also gives the *inner self* some elements to play with. Once we have acknowledged an image and seriously worked with it, even when we lay the work aside, further ramifications continue to suggest themselves, occasionally in thought and often in dreams.

THE LANGUAGE OF DREAMS

An alternative view of what is happening now

Your inner self uses a language quite different from the grammar of verbs and nouns in sentences. Initially, the signals you become aware of are the images in your dreams. To decode the language, start to reflect on these images, recall your dreams.

The best approach to analysis of a dream is to view it in the same way you look at a painting, listen to a song, or read a poem. Probably it is saying something meaningful with the most economical use of vivid, concentrated images possible. Consider those images, particularly the ones that recur frequently. They distill often paradoxical facts and emotions into a single statement. They are the elements of a language that comes straight from *your* depths.

It is not quite accurate to say they are the voice of the inner self, but they are closely related, and learning to read them is an important step in getting to know that unknown self.

Working with images from dreams as they emerge from the unconscious, relating to them, connecting them to the events and relationships in your conscious life causes you to sense an emerging pattern. Dreams disconnect some things and connect others in ways you would not consciously consider. If you pay close attention to your dreams, it begins to seem as if you are in a kind of dialogue with another. The dream is like a poem letter you receive which makes some comments on your concerns. Suddenly, it appears that certain figures seem to be recurring more frequently and acting in different ways in your dreams.

PAINTING AND TALKING WITH YOUR DREAM

It is useful to paint or draw the images of the dream to begin to get a sense of the underlying pattern which is emerging. Painting allows more of you to be involved than just your mind, but it also involves conscious choices in depicting and gives you (the conscious ego part of you) time to reflect on the image. Now you can give it a voice and *listen*. First, describe yourself as the image, e.g., "I'm an elevator in a tall building; I take people to the heights and the depths of the building down far into the subbasement. There's not much room in me; I can only take a few people at a time. My movement is always vertical; I have little to do with the horizontal. I run on only one track though, and I feel quite empty when I am not in use." Then you respond and the image answers. You are writing a dialogue.

Sometimes, describing yourself as the image is enough. The meaning, the analogy connecting the image to your everyday life, flashes through you; the linking can be dramatic, often bringing tears. The elevator image above was from one of my dreams when too much of my life was being lived in my work role as a psychotherapist. The same image, however, can have different meanings for different people. As in a poem, the meaning has to be established within the context of the whole dream and the allusions of the individual dreamer.

Each person has some few symbols with highly idiosyncratic meanings that recur almost like a signature, giving an originality in style and emotion to a dream series. A young, hippie girl at Esalen, with whom Fritz Perls once

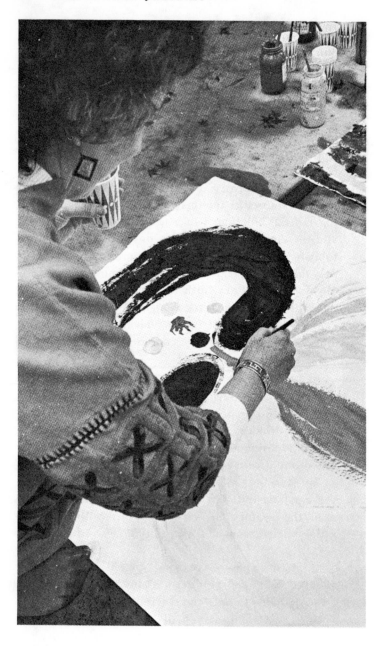

worked,voiced the same image: "I'm an elevator. I get used all the time. Men come into me and go out again..." Her surface pose as a sexually liberated woman covered a sense of being used, abandoned, and hurt. The dream brought this aspect to her attention and posed the question whether she chose to continue this or to risk acknowledging her need for great autonomy and making the change in lifestyle that would allow it.

Decoding the Dream

The Gestalt method of decoding dreams works mostly with the unconscious personal aspects of your situation or the functions that you do not consciously think of as your own. Using this method, you view everything that occurs in the dream as a part of yourself. When you have an unresolved conflict, the unconscious works at resolving it through dreaming. Each object in the dream, as well as each person and the setting itself, is an aspect of you that the dream is connecting in a different way than your conscious mind usually thinks.

To understand this suggested new wholeness, play the role, give a voice to each object or person in the dream. Look at your painting to decide the two images that are most unlike each other and create dialogue like writing a play, give a voice to each image *character* in turn. Getting them to come to an *understanding* can bring the deep issues of the dream to your conscious awareness.

Anna, whose family sculpture we looked at in the last chapter, had the following dream: "I am attending a conference in Hawaii. Something I have said has been misunderstood. Someone says I have many friends here, but I see Susan (a rival) and think to myself that I don't trust anyone here and I will stick to myself. A woman indicates she would like me to join the group for dinner at Pearl Harbor, a place not many tourists think to go. While at dinner, I notice a woman dressed in black and white whose hat is like a set of matches, eating at a table below ours. Later, I am removing leaves from an herb garden that has been neglected. They have lost all flavor and I throw them out."

She drew the dream and went on to write the following dialogue:

Anna to Pearl Harbor Restaurant: You're a very odd place to take nourishment, a symbol of infamy and sneak attacks.
Restaurant: You have come here and now I offer food.
Anna: Food for angry thoughts of past grievances.

Anna to Woman: Your hat is unusual and quite dangerous, it seems to me.
Woman (laughs): You think I might turn into a *hothead*, but I disguised this as a remarkable and elegant head cover.
Anna: A hat is for protection, but that is no protection for your head.
Woman: Don't be absurd. In the dark ages, hats were for protection, this is something else. I'm quite carefully dressed in black and white convictions and if I give the impression that my head is easily ignited, so much the better—elegant passion.
Anna: You seem to be mocking me using these things for show. I have deep convictions but I don't trivialize them and make a dangerous spectacle of myself.
Woman: We each have our self-righteous trip.

In the process of dialogue, Anna began to connect the current unacknowledged anger she was feeling toward her husband (under her Racket feeling of hurt at being misunderstood). She began to realize how she was taking nourishment for these feelings not from her present situation so much as from a place of past grievances where the issues of betrayal had once seemed very black and white. The volatile headgear was a vivid symbol of current anger which she had not previously identified.

Relating the Painting to the Dream

In your painting of the dream, you selected the important elements and related them to one another in placement on the paper. What did this add to your understanding? Do the kinds of images on the right differ from the left? The top from the bottom? Is there something in the center of your painting or is it empty? What do these positions mean to you? Is there any one object more dominant than the others? What would it do to the painting to shrink the dominant image and give a less conspicuous object more prominence?

In Anna's painting, she placed the hat of matches in the center which emphasized the central importance of the easily ignited or endangered head (thought processes). The herbs without flavor on the left side she thought of as past grievances which, she ruefully admitted, used to flavor her life but now had lost their flavor and she was ready to throw them out.

The object of this further play is simply that the conversation goes on. Tonight is another night and further dreams come. When you begin to work with your dreams this way, the character of your dreams changes and assumes a more purposeful direction. You notice more recurring symbols. A particular vocabulary of characters and symbols is building which begins to tap down into a source of meanings beneath the personal level of your life. Your dialogue with your dreams holds the possibility of gradually bringing you into relationship with the content deep inside your being and to symbols which foreshadow the wholeness towards which you are working. Relating to the images, connecting them to the events and relationships in your conscious life, causes a shifting of patterns. Anna's working with her dream of Pearl Harbor enabled her to see how past betrayals in her own life could inflame her current situation. Her next dreams continued with a restaurant theme but a different kind of *nourishment.*

Painting of a dream: *A bull and two cows are struggling to catch up with the family to which they belong. They are exhausted. A wise woman appears and makes cheese from their milk. She offers it to me but I am repulsed because of its vile smell. A girl like myself appears and tells me this is a very special food which I should accept.*

The painting emphasizes the primitive force and power of the instincts which can be transformed into a food to nourish the feminine development if she can overcome her repugnance and disgust. Elements in us which we consciously reject, hold a potential for our growth, a theme found frequently in fairy tales as well as dreams.

The total dream, coming as it does at a particular point in the dreamer's life, offers a comment on the present and frequently points a direction of development in the future. Lynn, a 25-year-old publishing house editor, had the following dream after the third session of her intensive treatment week:

Painting of a dream: *I have entered into a flirtation with a man. We are in a boat at sea and he drowns. I am helpless to rescue him.*

This dream frightened the dreamer and raised questions about her unconsciousness and irresponsibility in a current relationship, an alternative view and strong contrast to her conscious viewpoint.

I am beginning a trip to India. I join a family who are on a journey around the world. When we arrive in India, I am supposed to camp in a site this side of the Ganges River which my mother has described as beautiful and restful but when we arrive we find it is smelly, dangerous, and filled with thieves so we decide to go on. We are about to cross the Ganges River and I expect to encounter an unpleasant man described by my mother when she visited India years ago with my father. He guards the ferry and exploits his passengers. To my surprise I find the river is no more than a yard or so across for we are quite near the source. The man at the crossing simply questions me: do I want to cross? and I say yes, for my goal is a city on the other side, he guides me over. My mother seems to have joined us at this point and in bafflement says: "Things are not as they were."

Lynn was nonplussed by her dream. She had no religious interests and was turned off by both the Jesus-freaking of her younger sister and by the Eastern-style meditation/mysticism of her roommate. Yet this dream she felt had some sort of religious significance.

She said: "India is a very foreign place to me, a place of the rich and the very poor. It has produced many wise men and it is a place where wisdom is sought. I dream of it now because I seem to have begun a journey to foreign, unknown parts of myself. I am finding new feelings and conflicting thoughts within me. Yesterday and the day before when we worked on my relationship to my parents, I found out things I don't know what to do with, even how to think about them."

I suggested we look at the dreams with this in mind. She was on a journey but she was not alone, a family was there. She viewed them as healthy, happy, and adventurous; they were both a model of wholeness and a resource to her. The first encampment, the one urged on her by her mother, she rejected because she saw that it was not the place that her mother had imagined. This part of the dream Lynn connected to her view of her mother's role in life, a role of letting herself be exploited. The dream picture of a dangerous camp of thieves was an exaggeration of the awareness which had been growing in Lynn that early in her life her mother had placed herself in a position where her own development would be cut off and she had then rationalized her choice. She seemed to be self sufficient, invulnerable, and strong, a woman looked up to in her community and highly valued, yet her daughter knew her to be totally cut off from any real feelings of relatedness. She had no anger, no passion, no depth—she had been robbed of these and she denied her awareness. Lynn had been following her mother's footsteps.

Lynn went on with her exploration of the dream. The sacred river Ganges, the place of cleansing, had to be forded. For months prior to treatment, Lynn had been shaken by spells of unaccountable tears. They seemed fed by a river within her that would never end. Now she was close to the source. *Her* vision had been cleansed. She could see her goal, the sacred city in the distance. She could see the river was fordable and she simply had to ask to find the help she needed in crossing. She did not yet know who this masculine ferry keeper was within her but she knew she could count on his assistance. When she did, her mother would join her and things "would not be as they were."

This was a profoundly moving dream to both of us because it so clearly confirmed the work she had begun and the direction in which she would go.

Apart from the dialogues and written work with dreams, some art exercises can be used to deepen your experience of these aspects within. The art exercises which follow are designed to help you identify and contact two major inner realities: aspects of your sex that are most difficult for you to admit you own, and qualities of the opposite sex which you possess—the inner man in every woman, the inner woman in every man.

First, create a picture of how these parts relate to each other and to your goal of bringing to consciousness your creative inner self. In growing up, you probably disowned certain parts of your personality because they did not seem to fit with what other people expected of you and you enlarged those qualities that received approval, e.g., in America, we generally value personal openness, sociability, and material achievement so these qualities probably were reinforced in you as a child and gradually your contrary qualities, which weren't valued highly, were disguised and repressed. A lot of imagination and creative ability associated with the contrary qualities may have dried up in you as you became less

A Gestalt Doodle: *I began with no idea of what might develop, drew a line which turned into a man, then a tray appeared on which he was serving up a female satyr. She in turn developed a tray and is ready to serve someone else. It doesn't need a title; it's just fun to let go and see what comes.*

spontaneous. All of these disowned emotional components are called the *shadow* or *dark self*.

In addition, there is another unfamiliar part which might be called the inner woman in every man and the inner man in every woman. In a way that was similar to the development of your shadow side, you very likely repressed aspects of you and your experiences that did not correspond to the attributes your own sex is supposed to possess, e.g., a boy should be self-confident, assertive, logical. Qualities he regards as feminine, like tears, get pushed down, and the same thing happens with girls repressing their masculine intelligence or boisterousness or interest in mechanics.

As you begin to look for your inner self these parts push to be recognized. They appear in symbolic form in dreams (Anna's hotheaded woman was a shadow figure) but we can also consciously contact them through art as the following experiments suggest.

It seems when I get depressed, I am beating myself without mercy.

MEETING YOUR DARK SELF

Material you will need: a heap of old magazines, *Life* and *Look* used to be the richest source of supply for images, but any magazine that has pictures of human feelings and conditions will do. Scissors, gluestick, a pencil, scratch paper, and sturdy background paper.

First, note on the scratch paper all the characteristics of persons of *your own sex* who really get to you in a negative way, e.g., as a woman you may not be able to stand other women who are bitchy, controlling, whiney, manipulative, whatever, but specify the qualities that for you are the most obnoxious.

Go through the magazines and cut or tear out images that represent these qualities. When you have collected a sufficient pile, sift through and find those that really hold the essence for you and start your collage by gluing these in the center of your background sheet. Continue with the others.

When you have finished, spend some time looking at your production. You might pin it on your wall and live with it for a week before doing the next step, a dialogue. When you are ready, do a written exercise giving the collage a voice and writing the dialogue as it flows. It will flow as soon as you begin to consider this as an inner aspect which you have not given sufficient attention.

This experience can be illuminating. In one group, a minister's wife, middle-aged and beautiful but mild-looking, produced an hysterically funny collage which gave great prominence to a football helmeted and togged blond young woman, plus several images of Raquel Welch as a tough, mud-spattered, sexy roller derby winner. The following week, she tried to relate to this aspect within her and allowed it some room to act. She reported an astonishing success in a difference of opinion with her usually dictatorial husband. Another woman in the same group, but far more earthy, used a picture of a blond socialite whom she described as a phoney, ladylike manipulator. After acting *her* for a week, she had so many interesting reactions from her children, the plumber and the grocery clerk, she decided maybe there was some aspects of this symbol she could use validly after all.

CONTACTING THE INNER MAN IN EVERY WOMAN/THE INNER WOMAN IN EVERY MAN

The art exercise to relate to the inner elements of the opposite sex within you is the same as with the dark self, only here you select pictures related to both the very positive and the very negative feeling responses you have toward the opposite sex. *Playboy* and *Sports Illustrated* have many pictures involving plastic, sexual sterotypes, but also try to find pictures which capture your individual feelings.

Getting in touch with these inner opposites gives not only an uncomfortable sense of recognition of some of these patterns as they exist in you, but it may help you to view others whom you have despised in a more objective way. Owning and recognizing your own qualities gives you a fuller sense of who you are and releases energy that was tied up in keeping your self-image *clean*.

The guide in choosing a different direction

Once you begin to listen to the alternative points of view that your inner self suggests to you, you will find that you can carry on a dialogue with it about your life situations, problems, and possibilities. There are a number of processes that facilitate this conversation using your body, music, and art materials. You will find media provide different levels of experience.

Meditation, Painting, Music, and Mandalas

The many forms of meditation all propose to awaken a deeper consciousness. Most emphasize specific body positions, others involve movement. All involve stopping your ordinary activity and thought to allow an opportunity for different types of perception to emerge. Robert Ornstein, who has done research on the psychology of consciousness and meditation, uses an analogy, "You have to turn off the sun in order to see the stars." If you are not familiar with meditation, Shunryo Suzuki's *Zen Mind, Beginner's Mind* or Alan Watts' *The Essence of Alan Watts - Meditation* provides a start, but do not feel restricted to the presently popular Eastern techniques.

Basically, the first step is to release the body from its normal tensions. The easiest way to do this is to concentrate on your breathing. You can either sit comfortably erect or lie on the floor, flat on your back. Stay focused on your breath rhythm and count your exhalations. As thoughts come in, let them pass without getting involved with them. Let your attention be on your breathing. As you breathe out, envision the tensions of your body, the obstructions and static of your thoughts, draining away leaving an emptiness and receptivity. Hold the exhalation for a few seconds before taking a breath, then envision taking in, opening up to the energy and nourishment from without that you need. After awhile, the mental static which fills your mind during the day will clear away and you will be in a meditative state. Five minutes each day followed by a period of work with art will produce interesting progress in your use of art material.

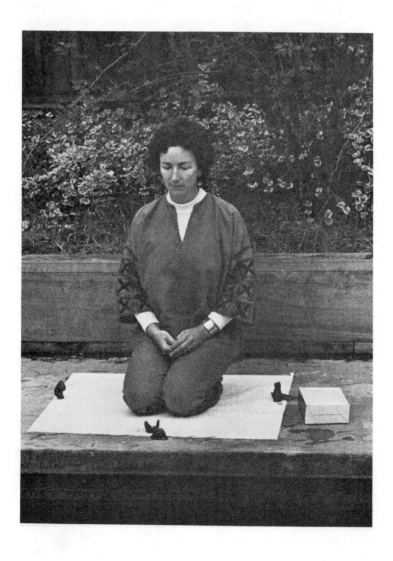

MEETING THE INNER OTHER IN PAINT

Material you will need: a large sheet of drawing paper and a set of colors—poster paints, water colors, felt-tip pens. Select a color that appeals to you without thought of what you are going to paint. Make a single mark on the paper of whatever size or shape seems right. Stop. Look at the colored portion and alternately at the shape of the non-colored portion. Allow yourself to sense what the next shape and color should be in relation to what is there. Proceed stopping each time between complete strokes to *look* and *listen.*

These paintings should be dated and collected without looking at them again for a period of several weeks. The development and progress in your choices and use of color shapes and symbols will be more apparent after you have several to refer to.

Louisa Jenkins, a renowned mosaicist whose art processes always include meditation, showed me a freeing-the-body painting exercise she uses to begin work. She spread newspapers on the floor of her studio and after performing relaxation exercises took two thick brushes, one in each hand, dipped them in a black india ink mixture, and standing over the paper bending from the waist, she began with both arms making large strokes much like calligraphy.

Music, carefully chosen, facilitates preparation. Louis Savary in *Passages: A Guide for Pilgrims of the Mind* writes of trance induction exercises for achieving altered states of consciousness. The basic reasons for wanting access to an altered state is to allow the perceptions and connections to emerge which are not available in ordinary everyday consciousness. In Savary's most recent book, *Music and Your*

Mind: Listening with a New Consciousness, he opens a further dimension, working with the multitude of mood and feeling potentialities in music. In my therapy groups and some workshops, I use cassette tapes he and Helen Bonney have developed which are available to the public from the Maryland Institute for Music and Consciousness. A typical selection of music is described in the suggested experience below.

Savary visualizes consciousness as a many-storied skyscraper. Its ground floor represents ordinary consciousness, the state of mind we use normally in thinking, feeling, problem-solving, remembering, and so on. But there are many higher and deeper levels of consciousness, whole floors devoted to creativity in art, music, invention, mathematics, deep memory, the collective unconscious and dreams, trans-personal, mystical and religious experiences. The building has an elevator and there are old and new techniques in addition to drugs, that can get you off the ground floor to bring you to the other levels. The techniques include biofeedback, sensory deprivation, mind-control, Zen and Transcendental Meditation, and self-hypnosis. Most people, however, seldom go beyond the mind's first floor.

It is one thing to know that these levels exist and wish to explore them, it is another to get there, and still another to know what to do when you get there.

This is my loneliness. I'm on the edge of a gaping hole, a deep pit in the middle of a desert.

AN ALTERED STATE OF CONSCIOUSNESS
WITH GUIDED IMAGERY

What you will need: a quiet room, a stereo phono-graph and music which has pleasant-feeling possi-bilities (Ravel, *Daphis and Chloe;* Brahms, *Symphony No. 1 in C (3rd Movement);* Respighi, *The Pines of Rome;* Debussy, *Girl with the Flaxen Hair*), any music at all that you'd like to feel more deeply.

Relaxation. To feel relaxed is to feel weightless, that the body's muscles are in balance, neither pushing nor pulling. If you are familiar with any relaxation techniques—Zen or Transcendental Meditation, childbirth relaxation exercises, be-havior modification, mind control or self-hypnosis —and you find that they help you, by all means use them. In this exercise, comfort is essential. Relax in the way that feels best to you.

One method is to become aware of the various parts of your body relaxing in turn, first your toes, then the foot with its arch, instep, ball, heel, ankle —let go of all effort, rest—the legs, the hands, arms, shoulders, the abdomen, chest, throat, facial muscles, and eyes. It helps to use certain key phrases that eventually become deeply associated with the state of relaxation and trigger it the next time you wish to relax with much less effort—*let go* in a quiet tone of voice. Try to maintain an even rhythm in your breathing. Develop a regular pattern for bringing on this quietly balanced state and practice it often. The more complete the relaxation is, the deeper will be the listening state. In first starting out, it may take up to a half hour to reach a deep state of relaxation, but with practice it will be possible in a few minutes.

Concentration. Once the body is relaxed, your mind is ready to concentrate. This involves focusing your mind on an object as simply and as quietly as you would a camera lens—a flower, a burning candle—and become quietly absorbed in it. Do not analyze, describe, or define it, but receive it in such a way that you can see it in every detail even with your eyes closed. Later, your mind will be able to create its own objects. Every time you exercise your mind power, you are preparing for a fuller listening experience. Many teachers recommend sounding a word or syllable. Humming or intoning a single note and holding it sets up a vibration which affects the entire body and helps it to respond.

The Induction. The goal of this beginners' induction is a summer meadow, a place that you remember having enjoyed and would like to enjoy again now listening to some restful music. Begin by visualizing yourself standing at a doorway. You open a door and before you in the soft twilight mist is a winding mountain path. As you start out with each step, count slowly from ten to zero. At each step, suggest to yourself that the mist will soon disappear and you will sense your warm, sunlit meadow. When you reach zero, allow yourself to feel the change with your feet, your skin, your hearing, and let the music lead you into different experiences in this meadow.

When the music has ended, remain quiet for a minute or so, then suggest to yourself that as the music has ended, you are ready to return to normal consciousness, you will count from three to zero. When you reach zero, you will open your eyes and be in your normal state, fully rested and alert and feeling deeply satisfied. You may want to review the insights gained during the session and tell yourself you will be able to recall them easily whenever you wish.

The exercise above is a beginning. Once you enter the suggested deep state of relaxation, you can begin to listen to music in a new way with your total awareness. You will normally never entirely leave ordinary consciousness, you will continue to hear doors slam and street sounds. Yet your everyday awareness will grow less important as the music itself begins to engage you on other levels of consciousness, for example, memories and dreams, insight, self-evaluation, and creativity.

Almost everyone enters these areas of the mind at one time or another, but few live familiarly with them in the same way that composers, poets, and inventors do. Your mind is able to contain many ideas and experiences at the same time. Music seems to acquire colors, shapes, motion, even taste and scent, and to generate greater levels of emotional intensity and depth when you listen in a state of heightened awareness. Melodies, harmonies, and rhythms open up meanings within you, you see more ways to look at a problem, an idea, a person.

You must practice to reach the deeper levels of altered consciousness, but the above exercise will almost invariably induce a light trance which is characterized by being hyper-aware of the music. As you develop familiarity with this process, you can program guided fantasy trips. John Stevens has a number of excellent fantasy exercises in his book *Awareness*, a resource book for exercises which increase the awareness of various senses and different levels of experience in relationships with other people.

One which I use quite frequently in workshops is: Imagine you are out for an evening stroll in a town with which you are familiar and feel safe. As you walk, you pass by a street that is unknown to you but seems interesting. You turn and walk down the left side of the street until you come to a deserted store. As you pass the window, an abandoned object in it catches your eye and you draw closer. Look at it closely, let yourself become the object and imagine your history. Now go back to being you and continue your walk. When the exercise is ended, I suggest that the participants paint a picture of the object.

In discussing these paintings, I find they almost always have a symbolic connection with some experience unfinished or left behind in the individual's life. I ask each person to identify with his painting and describe himself as it. Each is free to discuss his painting as much or as little as he chooses. Others present can make a comment but in the first person and present tense also, thereby owning projections rather than interpreting for another. For example, one man described himself as a clock, "I'm wooden, run down and rusty." Another man looking at the same painting added, "I'm a trifle out of date, but my works are in good order and, with a bit of cleaning out and regular attention, I can function quite well." Each man spoke from and referred to his own emotional feeling.

Often in these fantasies, you will discover the presence of opposite or opposing values and interests. One way to deepen your understanding of these polarities is to meditate on them as you construct a mandala to express the interplay between the elements.

The Mandala. A circle motif in its manifold combinations with the square is one of the great symbols of wholeness. It is commonly found in dreams and also throughout the world in the art of every culture; it is universal in nature. The construction of a mandala involves and satisfies a need for order. It is both a process and a product of meditation. In it you can explore the intrinsic relationship between darkness and light, evil and good, or whatever opposites you want to pair. The yin-yang symbol epitomizes this. When one aspect, yang, the light, reaches its greatest strength, the dark power of yin is born within its depths: "...for night begins at midday when yang breaks up and begins to change into yin."

Jung described constructing a mandala as an expression of a self-healing process through which the psyche maintains its sanity and nurtures its own growth. This symbol, he said, finally contains the "innermost god-like essence of man." It stands for the deity as well as the self since it reflects the image of the godhead in the unfolded creation in nature and in man.

You are not likely to have such lofty thoughts immediately since you are more concerned with the opposites, e.g., you love and resent your children at the same time, or you want to be powerful and independent at the same time you feel yielding, soft, and needy. In order for the process to be effective you must begin where you are.

In creating a mandala you might try it first with paint but you should feel free to make other choices—some people dance them. Jung, when he wanted to reach his creative source not only painted but also played with stones as building blocks. Use whatever material appeals to you. Some illustrations are provided, but *your* mandala will develop in your relating to the particular polarities, opposites that you are attempting to reconcile and understand in your life.

The one essential element to a mandala is a *center.* Symmetry and cardinal points brought into relationship with one another around this center are basic elements but they will vary according to the nature of what is depicted. The mandala will essentially be a vehicle for concentrating your mind so you can relate to apparent contradictions in order to reach a deeper, more inclusive sense of your inner center, the source of your energy, your inner self. For this reason it is important that you take great care and concentration. First find a quiet room or a natural setting, then choose the issue you want to explore, one of the following perhaps.

MANDALA POSSIBILITIES

1. Your day and your night, the different aspects of you that come into awareness with the dawn, the activity of the day, the transition of dusk into evening, and finally the part of you that comes into being with the night.

2. The present year, or your life span from birth to death, or the particular period of your life you are in now.

3. Your body, top and bottom, right and left sides, front and back. Feel and think out your attitudes towards each part.

4. The inner experience of you and your outer relationships with others or of the relationship between your masculine and feminine aspects, your thinking and feeling, and any other division you are aware of.

5. Make a mandala with another person. First, in talking, explore your differences and their relationship to one another; then, in painting, find the colors and symbols to express how each of you experiences yourself in relationship to the other.

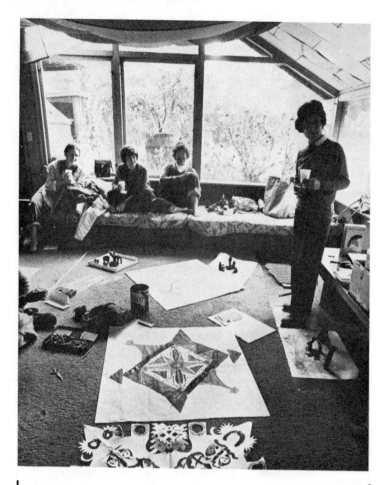

Now that you have chosen your issue, center yourself by letting the cares and concerns of the day drop away, concentrate your conscious mind to develop an image of your center. You might close your eyes and envision a blank piece of paper and simply wait. The image which comes might be a flame, a star, a stone, a circle, whatever. When it appears, make that the center of your construction. Now consider the opposites that you are going to work with.

Stay with this as long as necessary to find and simplify the most basic qualities of these opposites. You want to develop a symbolic awareness. You may have begun with the rhythm of a day and a night in your life but when you symbolize them you may find they extend to a basic statement and awareness of life and death. Go with your awareness to as many levels as occur, then again search for the essential symbols to express what you have found. Add these to your mandala, relating them in their dynamic polarity to your existing center.

The dialogue mandala is particularly useful with your marriage partner. So often it is possible to implicitly assume your wife or husband has to think as you do or feel as deeply about something as you do, or you are not understood. Another possibility is that you each need the other to be very much as he/she is to provide a balance and a tension for your growth as an individual. For instance, in doing this exercise, my husband who is quite concrete and specific in his thinking and goal directed, represented himself in the center of the mandala as a diamond-edged, multicolored star. I am more of a goal drifter but oriented to energy and *seeing what wants to*

happen, so I represented myself as a flame sparking out from between and around his edges, a fairly accurate reflection of the problems and richness we hold for one another.

Learning what you are, how you function inside yourself and with those persons closest to you, you are by that very awareness changing yourself. You are becoming more responsive and responsible for the growth of your inner wholeness, finding your inner center which now guides the integration of all that you are. However, there is one further step which involves taking an overview of your whole life span, and for this it is useful to look at life stories, your own and others.

Myths, life scripts and your own transformation

Myths are man's attempt to answer *why?* Why are things the way they are and how did they get started? Marie Louise von Franz, a Jungian analyst who has delved deeply into the figures, persons and patterns in fairy tales, suggests that ultimately these tales, too, all tell the same story of man's journey and the different archetypal elements with which he must come to terms. Your interest in looking at these universal stories now is to identify whether they have something specific to say to you about your individual life story.

Eric Berne, in developing Transactional Analysis, outlined a typology in his versions of myths and fairy tales to explain some of the common forms of personal disturbance he observed. He said there are only a limited number of possible ways to live your life, and they have all been capsulized in myth and fairy tale. In working with a patient, he found it useful to relate the patient's life to a coherent story which has survived for hundreds or thousands of years because of its universal appeal to the primitive layers of the human mind. This, at the least, gave him a feeling of working from a solid foundation and, at best, very precise clues as to what needed to be done to avoid a bad ending. An amusing and rueful example he developed is "Sleeping Beauty or Waiting for Rigor Mortis." The story is one of the many myths about a magic sleep. Remember Brunhild left sleeping on the mountain with a ring of fire around her which only the hero Siegfried can penetrate? These myths all contain some of the same elements: a woman caught by the evil spell of another, a long period of sleep cut off from contact with the ordinary world, a hero who overcomes the obstacles or simply comes at the right time, and an awakening.

In "Sleeping Beauty " an angry fairy says that Briar Rose, Sleeping Beauty, will prick her finger with a spindle when she is 15 and will fall down dead. Another fairy commutes this to 100 years of sleep. When she is 15, she does prick her finger, immediately falls asleep, and at the same time everything and everyone else in the castle also falls asleep. During the hundred years, many princes try to reach her, but none succeed until the time is up at last and a prince arrives who finds Briar Rose, kisses her, she wakes, and they fall in love. At the same time, everyone else takes up exactly where they left off as though nothing had happened. The princess herself is still 15 and not 115.

The problem for a present-day heroine living this life story or script is that everything and everybody cannot be unchanged after a lapse of so many years. *This* is the illusion on which the script is based, that modern Rose be 15 years old again instead of 30, 40, or 50 when she wakes up, and that she and the Prince will have a whole lifetime ahead of them. It is hard to tell a real life Rose that princes are younger men and by the time they reach her age, they have become kings, settled down, and are usually much less interested.

This script is also known as "Frigid Woman" because the woman acting it out has often bought the notion that she should not feel sexual, that part of her is sleeping. There is usually an antiscript in which it would be okay if she married the right person, i.e., the Prince with the Golden Apples. A practical problem occurs if she does find the Prince with the Golden Apples. She may feel outclassed and find fault by playing "Blemish" to bring him down to her level, or if she settles for less—the Prince with the Silver Apples, or even ordinary McIntoshes from the grocery store—she will feel cheated and take it out on him while still keeping an eye out for the Golden One.

This script is important because a great many people, one way or another, spend a lifetime waiting for the Prince, the Rescuer, the right job, right opportunity, whatever, instead of waking up to the reality that they individually are responsible for making the condition or quality of their own lives.

Berne s typology of myths and fairy tales pictures the protagonist as blocking, evading, or fearing growth. His treatment aims to recover the original growth impulses, but Berne did not take the next step. He did not identify the myth of the person who achieves wholeness.

A model exists: the journey of the Hero constitutes a universal heritage of mankind. We are probably most familiar with stories like John Bunyan's *Pilgrim's Progress*, or Bible heroes like Joseph who was abandoned by his brothers in jealousy and became the King's advisor in Egypt, or the Greek heroes and heroines, Hercules, Ulysses, Jason of the Golden Fleece, Psyche, Persephone. But all cultures have similar Hero journeys: Beowulf in the Anglo-Saxon, Kiovick in the Eskimo, Parsifal in the German.

Basically, the story starts with the hero in a known but stagnant place. Things were once good in his land but now a sense of blight has taken over and some reparation or restoration has to take place. This he undertakes by starting the journey to the unknown and thus begins a time of trials: he meets his opposites, overcomes dragons and other terrors while keeping his wits about him. Mastering the first trial, he develops strength for the next and sometimes gets a magic potion or amulet from the conquest that will stand him in good stead in later difficulties. There are always several more to come. In the process of his journey, he undergoes a transformation, and when he returns to his land, the missing element is restored and he is recognized as the Hero, the one who completed the task. The land is healed.

My view of the hero is not as the exceptional man (although at present there may be relatively few self-actualizing men) but rather as that unfolding potential in every person which can be unblocked. Every person undertakes a journey when he begins to consciously accept responsibility for his own choices. What shall I do with today? What shall I do with my life? How can I deal with my anxiety, aggression, and hostility? How shall I meet these feelings in others? How can I use my sexuality fully and creatively? What does personal integrity demand? What meaning is there in the word *God?* Choices in answer to questions like these orient the beginning quest.

Your story is largely determined by the situation into which you are born, and you stagnate until a certain degree of consciousness awakens usually through a crisis—a death, divorce, loss of an important goal—or perhaps the recognition that you just don't fit your context, something you would never have chosen. You are forced down into what feels like emptiness and often despair. After a time you begin to grope in the darkness, looking for some way out. Perhaps you enter therapy, perhaps you do it on your own. But with this first step you begin the upward ascent. You begin your journey.

Jeremy, the young lawyer whose family sculpture we considered, was thinking of divorce until it occurred to him that his sense of not fitting was much broader than just his relation to his wife. The pervasiveness of his sense of boredom and lack of meaning initially felt to him like a tight prison with no way out. Paradoxically, that is the turning point. Only by realizing the full darkness and emptiness he had been avoiding, could he begin to ask the right questions. Why am I living the way I am, what are the possible choices I did not acknowledge, what were their costs, is it too much to pay to become my *own man?*

The time of trials takes you through peaks and valleys of feeling, down and up until you reach a point at which everything is seen in a new light. You then become conscious of the underlying purposiveness in your life, particularly of the darkness that you regarded as evil. If Jeremy hadn't fallen into a depression, he would have continued to exist half alive. So the evil, the depression, was the way out. Some describe this recognition as satori, others as enlightenment, still others as individuation. It is not an end point. The journey goes on.

One such Hero tale, cited by analysts Elizabeth Howes and Sheila Moon in *Man the Choicemaker* is that of Sir Gawain and Lady Ragnell. Gawain, one of King Arthur's finest knights, in order to save the life of his beloved king, agreed to marry a loathsome lady with a hideous face and great twisting eyes. She seemed to be enormously greedy and fat and sat hunched on her horse like a great bale of straw. Gawain kept his promise although the court shuddered with horror. On their wedding night, Gawain kissed her and afterward wept in agony, but at that instant, Ragnell, who had been enchanted, was freed and became her young and beautiful self—but for only half each twenty-four hour period. Gawain must choose, she said, did he want her beautiful by night and repellant by day, or the other way around? Gawain answered, "With you is the greatest suffering, and you alone must choose what you are most able to bear." With this final sacrifice, the enchantment completely lifted. What he offered up was enormous, the humiliating sacrifice of his own desires for the sake of the Round Table and its safety. What he received back was more—his king's life preserved, the security of the Round Table, and an unexpected love.

In a group discussing this tale of sacrifice and redemption and making it more personally relevant, one man might remark all choice inevitably involves sacrifice. In order to develop any relationship with another, some personal autonomy has to be given up. Another person's first thought is how preconceptions have to be let go in the process of creating an original work. A third comments that for the sake of psychological growth, favorite self images and defenses have to be laid aside.

A theme gradually develops of how we shun and are reluctant to relate to the darker aspects of ourselves because we are so unwilling to give up our favorite points of view and our onesided images. But all sacrifice is not redemptive! Look at the people who play martyr and victim games. Clearly there are two kinds of sacrifice, one egocentric in its manipulative desire to be praised and loved, and the other a letting go *to* something which is of greater value. In the tale, the greater value was the life of the king and the security of the Round Table, that great symbol of wholeness.

Excerpts from a journal:
3 February 1972: *I am experiencing another self that I have not been in touch with. I feel the greatest need to SEE that other self and make contact.*

8 May 1972: *I have entered the valley of the Shadow of Death. I am feeling despair, not that I can't go on, but yes that I must go on. The tree in the foreground is living but the dead tree in the distance tells me that I am coming to a place where something in me must die so that something else can be born.*

22 December 1972: *Everything is blue in this painting. I have moved from a world of red hot heat into water. I feel tranquil and peaceful. The man inside and the woman inside me are together on the raft and moving towards the horizon where the edge of the sun appears. It seems to me that the Sun which can't be fully seen yet is centered on this page and is my own wholeness.*

Each participant now considers for himself alone, either in writing or using art media to focus his attention. Who or what is Ragnell to me? To what aspect of my life does she correspond? What feels grotesquely deformed and hideous in myself that I must relate to? One woman may find her reflections leading in the direction of a current struggle she is facing between choosing to stay in a stable and good but endlessly tepid marriage or giving it up for a new relationship which promises to be richly creative. She does not wish to hurt her husband whom she genuinely cares for but she does not want to lose this new meaning. What is she to do? Shall she renounce the new and struggle with the old? Shall she work with the new meanings only inside herself? What is the larger value which needs to be rescued? Another person might find his Ragnell to be a long buried hostility that has at last been uncovered. How should he relate to it? Hold on to it, let go of it, express it, work with it in some other way? Each person struggling with these questions has to risk his individual decisions. He has to renounce his old dependence on outer authority but his self respect and personal strength grows.

There are two ways to work with myths. One used by the Guild for Psychological Studies in San Francisco starts with an actual myth, e.g., the Legends of the Grail. Usually two leaders work with the texts and the group in a Socratic dialogue that enables each participant to take the story inward and relate it to the personal content of his life. Later, in working alone with art materials, each person develops the symbols most meaningful for him personally. Sharing these in a later group session deepens the experience for all.

The following method is a way of discovering your personal myth. I use it with both individuals and groups.

WRITING YOUR MYTH

Write the story of your life as a myth. What is your mythic name? What was the event or crisis that started you on your journey? Who are your companions and how did you meet? You might personify your dark self as well as your inner man or inner woman. What was the land like from which you started? Where did you go? Who and what did you encounter? Then what happened?

Cassie, an ex-nun living alone and working at a bookkeeping job that in no way reflected her abilities, took no initiative in establishing a social life and put down attempts by others to get to know her. From her dreams and fantasies, she identified a cast of characters within her: a crying baby she despised; a small, red, angry child; a critic analyst also known as the executioner; and a totally inept mediator who was the designated leader but who felt helpless when the others fought. I had her imagine them starting out on a journey together, what they would each bring, and how they would manage various obstacles.

By understanding her myth, she found that the crying child actually had a strong ability to judge what possibilities and situations would feel right for all of the group to explore, she did not cry at all when interested and taken care of. The angry red child was male, had independence, strength, and more than a streak of the adventurer in him; he scouted territory and found and made bridges over dangerous chasms. The critic was nasty but also a very good computer-navigator and by the end had developed his own brand of vinegary humor, a quite tolerable companion indeed. We were now able to look for the strengths in her. She could acknowledge them as her own.

Now you have some direction. You have formed some images of the place you stand and from where you start. You have some navigation instruments, your dreams and active imagination, and from your inner explorings you have begun a tentative map. You need time alone now to discover your inner aspects, how you need to nourish them and continue your journey. A time to be inwardly attentive is essential to the growth of those small beginnings, the gathering together of meaning.

As one who makes the inward journey, you come to see outer reality more accurately, unscreened and free from distortions of your projections and wants. You know you can find and react to all sorts of symbols, from inside as in your dreams and from outside in the outer events and persons who enter your life. Broader than that, you can find your connection to the very cosmos itself. Recent discoveries in astronomy, physics, biology, paleontology, and geology show a complex web of relationships between ourselves, our planet, our solar system, our galaxy, with one another and the universe that gave birth to us all. Just as when you looked at the collected wisdom in myths for parallels to understand your own journey towards wholeness, you can also find similar parallels in the objective scientific story of the formation of simple chemical compounds, the growth of organic molecules, the development of living tissue to the capacity for self aware-ness. Von Ditfurth in his *Children of the Universe*, Teilhard de Chardin in *The Phenomenon of Man*, Loren Eiseley, Fred Hoyle, Rachel Carson—these are a few of the scientists who place our inward journey in the wonderous context of a continuing story. You alone, however, can relate the two worlds, inner and outer, choosing, persevering, bringing together many opposites, sacrificing the self images that act as barriers to understanding. And nothing feeds this process so much as creative work. Although I use art forms in therapy, my aim is not solely to point to these as potentially fulfilling pursuits in themselves but as tools to open up for consideration the many possibilities of the inner life that have not been explored and can be expressed in creative action.

Susanne K. Langer says it well in an essay on "The Growing Center of Knowledge":

> Only a small part of reality for a human being is what is actually going on; the greater part is what he imagines in connection with the sights and sounds of the moment.... This is not to say his life is a dream, his world a fantasy or any such pseudo-philosophical thing. It means that his world is bigger than the stimuli that surround him and the measure of it is in the reach of his steady and coherent imagination. An animal's environment consists of things that act on his senses....a human being's world hangs together. Its events fit into each other; no matter how devious their connections, in one big framework of time and space.... The world is something human. (Langer, pp. 145–46)

That getting a sense of "how my world hangs together" is essential. You need to give yourself time for the thoughtful going inward, time for a deeper connection with your surroundings and senses as well as the imaginative consideration of possible options, the wonderful "what if's" you can consider, then choose, in developing and allowing your multifaceted self to be.

Maps and Charts ## II.

THE CREATIVE PROCESS

Creativity lies in the discovery of unsuspected links. Before the new possibilities emerge, however, there is usually a period of massive discomfort. In my experience as a psychotherapist, this crisis and feelings of anger, pain, boredom, and self-dissatisfaction that originally brings a person into psychotherapy, often correspond to the first stage of a profoundly creative process. The individual able to proceed beyond this stage will achieve greater awareness and solutions to the personal problems that confront him.

Clearing away the obstacles to this process consists largely of helping the individual to discover his present autonomy and unacknowledged power. Transactional Analysis is one of the tools used to guide to this discovery. TA offers quick, effective methods for identifying the decisions an individual has made in the light of his early life situation, decisions that currently distort his perceptions and ability to meet his present needs.

In applying the framework of TA to their problems, some people find the gimmicky language and apparent oversimplification obstructive. Initially this is how it seemed to me when I was studying with Eric Berne 20 years ago. His succinct restatement of the essence of Freudian theory, group dynamics, and what we then knew of social psychology, I recognized as elegant if unorthodox, but the feelings and emotions of the client did not seem to matter enough. Something was missing in the gamey *nothing but* explanations of behavior. A woman may play "If It Weren't for You" to hide her doubts of her own ability and reluctance to accept the discipline of a career. Defining the game helps her to face these issues; however, it may block seeing her behavior as proceeding from any other level of meaning, e.g., the interplay of values between her creative power and her destructive anger, that within her which pushes for transformation.

The Gestalt approach of Fritz Perls added an essential dimension to my knowledge—the living here and now experience of the client with his full feeling complexity, the various elements within his person warring and struggling to be recognized. TA and Gestalt combine to form powerful tools for understanding behavior. The woman in a Gestalt experience of her game "If It Weren't for You" enacts her projection of her husband's constraint, then her talent struggling to be free. She feels strongly this polarization within her and, in attempting to form a bridge between them, she uncovers and owns the value they represent.

What was now missing was something I had not previously included in psychology—the *meaning* in a person's life, the sense of being more than we can account for that struggles for expression in what we aspire to be and do. Jung's writings gave some indication of the importance of this *meaning*, but I didn't immediately realize the *means* for understanding the more than was here. During Jungian analysis with Joseph Wheelwright, I discovered art methods with collage brought me into touch with aspects of self which had a reality beyond the confines which I had previously thought of as *myself*. The process I was beginning is one common to artists, musicians, scientists, actors, but also to preschoolers absorbed in finger painting and high schoolers struggling to write a theme paper.

There is a phase of uneasiness, of sensing that something wants to happen, then an exploring and manipulating of some material, finding out about the elements of it, the possibilities, combinations and patterns, ways of doing and using. There are phases of frustration and a need to get away from it and turn our conscious thoughts to something else, but we keep being drawn back. Suddenly, there it is. The elements have come together in a pattern and we are almost flooded with what wants to come out, what wants to be expressed. We *see* what we had not seen before.

There seems to be an aspect within each of us that, if given sufficient material, will begin to organize in patterns that express something of its otherwise unseeable self. By analogy, this is like scattering iron filings on a paper over a magnet. Each iron particle reacts to the magnetic field, becoming magnetized by induction, attracting or repelling the other nearby granules, all of which become organized into a pattern corresponding to the magnetic field of the underlying magnet. We then see a pattern on the paper which represents intense magnetization, the lines of force of the otherwise invisible field. This aspect within us serves as a magnetic field, developing materials in patterns of creative purpose.

The work we do with material and thought provides the stimulus. Then when we let go with our efforts, the influence of the creative field begins to intensify. The preparation we do provides the basic elements with which the creative field plays. Our creative aspect selects those elements which correspond most closely to its own patterns and contributes insight to our problem. The incubation stage during which the creative field develops and is expressed without conscious manipulation can last from a few seconds to many years. Some of the patterns which recur time after time correspond remarkably to universal symbols that are found in myths, fairy tales, art, and literature of all cultures. They also recur in the dreams and art processes of the person looking inward at his own consciousness. They are partially what Jung identified as the archetypes, inherited experiences unconscious in the present individual. Recently astronomers, paleontologists, physicists and other scientists have discovered similar patterns in the cosmos, linking processes occurring in the formation of the stars to the formation of organic molecules through the development of our own self-reflective awareness. When we experience and try out new meanings we are deeply involved with the very stuff of the cosmos.

The growth process of connecting with all that we are capable of being resumes when we stop limiting ourselves and unlock some of the energy used to do the limiting. I consider the theories of TA, Gestalt, and Jungian psychology to be integrally related. They are like charts and maps. TA can clear the ground and provide much of the preparation, Gestalt unblocks the emotional power, and Jungian thought provides a sense of direction.

Transactional Analysis (TA) began when Eric Berne observed a man change his tone of voice, his facial expression, and his gestures. In the course of a relatively few minutes, he was a whining little boy, then switched to acting like a stern judgmental parent even to shaking his fist. Finally he changed to a reflective adult computing some changes in his business that had to be made. Berne concluded that each of us operates from three basically different ego states. These are characterized by different feelings, actions, types of decisions, body postures, and gestures.

Parent: *When I am acting like I once experienced one of my parents act.*

Adult: *When I am objective and responding to "here and now."*

Child: *When I am emotionally feeling as I used to feel as a child.*

When in a *Parent* state of mind the person embodies actual sets of feelings, values, maxims, and judgments that he once experienced coming from one of his parents. He may literally use the tone of voice or gestures that his parent used to put over his point of view.

When in a *Child* ego state he is operating with the feelings, drives, and needs that he actually experienced in childhood.

In the *Adult* ego state he is present-centered, in touch with the situation in which he finds himself. He is making decisions and acting with a real here and now response to what the situation calls for. This is in contrast to the Parent response which characteristically is a should or ought type of judgment failing to compute relevant information that had not been available or would have been ignored by the original parent. The Adult state response differs from the Child in computing consequences rationally rather than acting from a feeling or need response.

In growing up, each child makes *Decisions* that largely determine the kind of life he is going to lead. These are made in response to his experiences but particularly in response to certain messages he receives from his parents. Bear in mind that each parent has three ego states too, so some of their messages may come from a hurt, confused, inadequate, or frightened Child that has limited them and which they pass on to their children.

Injunctions: Don'ts and Dos

Injunctions are comprised of all the messages received from the Child part of the parents. These messages tend to be the *Don'ts* and are sometimes deadly, e.g., *Don't be (Don't exist)*, from the woman who did not want a child and viewed it as an interference with what she did want. Sometimes the parent has wanted a child of the opposite sex, and the child gets the message *Don't be a girl*, or *Don't be a boy*. Often when the parent has failed to achieve something he/she wanted, the child gets the message, *Don't be you (Be my ideal self)*. The messages are given verbally and nonverbally, directly and indirectly, e.g., *I'm cold; go put on your sweater, Johnny. You're not hungry yet; you're just tired*, eventually gets translated: *Don't feel what you feel; feel what I feel.*

Sometimes when tears and anger are not acceptable, the child gets the message, *Don't feel* or *Don't be a child.* Occasionally something in the parent is threatened if the child is too talented or too successful and *Don't make it* or *Don't be important* are sent. Other messages are *Don't be well* or *Don't be sane* and sometimes just *Don't* (*Whatever you're doing, stop it*).

From the Parent ego state of the parent comes other messages about what would please the parent, make the child acceptable, and what behaviors will be rewarded. TA calls attention of any kind *stroking;* the child can work for positive (approval) or negative (punishment) strokes, the latter on the theory that any attention is better than none. The Parent instructions tend to be worded as such: *Work hard; Be a lady; Make good grades; Be strong; Be unselfish; Be obedient: Be seen but not heard; Be popular; Be kind; Be perfect.*

Just as a child easily learns the native language of his country and this language shapes his perceptions, things he recognizes as important, each family has it's own emotional language which determines the Injunctions and which emotional experience the child will recognize as important. A child whose early experience of women is bossy and domineering will later be more highly aware of bossy domineering traits in women than another whose experience of women was of a gentle and submissive mother.

Decisions

While the messages received from parents make up the child's *Injunctions,* his *Decisions* are made to buy or not to buy the Injunctions based on the kind of stress in which he finds himself and the ways he sees to get strokes he needs to survive in this given place and this given time. The problem comes when these early Decisions have been carried forward and the present day situation is not the same, e.g., the man has physical power and freedom to determine his choices that the child did not possess but he can still be acting out of an ego state that feels powerless.

Some of the problematic Decisions the child can make are:

> *I'll show you, even if it kills me.*
>
> *If things don't go right, I'll kill myself.*
>
> *I'll get you, even if it kills me.*
>
> *I'll do the things the other sex does. . . and I'll be lonely.*
>
> *I'll show you I can be a boy/girl.*
>
> *I'll never really make it.*
>
> *I'll succeed but I won't enjoy it.*
>
> *I'll never let anyone know my real feelings (I'll hide my feelings).*
>
> *I'm no good.*
>
> *It does not pay (work) to put myself first.*

Anna's situation used in family sculpting illustrates the interplay between Injunctions, Decisions, and Redecisions. Adult Redecisions based on current reality and not programmed by the past can be made when the underlying pattern of Injunctions, Decisions, Rackets, Games, and Scripting is apparent.

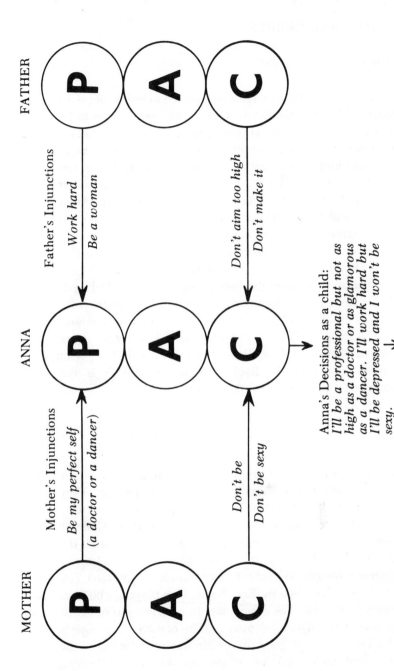

MOTHER

P

A

C

Mother's Injunctions

Be my perfect self
(a doctor or a dancer)

Don't be

Don't be sexy

ANNA

P

A

C

FATHER

P

A

C

Father's Injunctions

Work hard

Be a woman

Don't aim too high

Don't make it

Anna's Decisions as a child:
*I'll be a professional but not as
high as a doctor or as glamorous
as a dancer. I'll work hard but
I'll be depressed and I won't be
sexy.*

Anna's Redecisions as an adult:
*I'll be a sexy woman and a
highly competent professional.*

Rackets

Rackets in TA terminology refer to a person's chronic negative stereotyped feeling reaction to stress. Some people seem to be chronically angry, others depressed, others confused. A Racket gets started in the early family situation when one or more feelings are highly unacceptable. In Anna's family it was not O.K. to feel either sexy or to feel angry, so instead of having those forbidden feelings when they were called for, Anna would feel sad and powerless which was acceptable and even got some stroking in the form of attention.

Racket feelings are substitutes for the true feeling called for in a situation. When the true feeling is identified, it calls for an action to achieve the underlying need. The feeling is then discharged and the person moves on to meet the next emerging situation. He is not hung up with any particular feeling. A Racket feeling on the other hand is never on target so the real need is not identified and taken care of. The person continues to collect the Racket feeling because it is not discharged; it does not meet the underlying need.

Games

Games, as defined by TA, are ways of interacting with others (or in one's own head) that end up with Racket feelings. They start with an ostensibly straight message to the other person's Adult but this contains a secret message to the other's Child or Parent state. The secret message is responded to and the initiator collects his *old familiar feeling*.

One of the easiest games to recognize is "Why Don't You Yes But" first described by Eric Berne: One player, who is *it*, presents a problem. The others start to present solutions each beginning with, *Why don't you*. . . The one who is *it* objects with a *Yes, but*. . . A good player can stand off the rest of the group indefinitely until they all give up, whereupon *it* wins.

The ostensible purpose, an Adult quest for information, contains a secret message from the Child, *I'm inadequate to meet this situation*, designed to hook the other person's sage Parent, anxious to dispense wisdom, which is exactly what *it* wants since her object is to confound these Parents one after the other. As the game ends, all those who offered advice are dejected, having failed to help and *it* has proved the point that her problem is really insoluble which makes it possible for her to indulge herself in her Racket feeling of depression and self-pity.

The real feeling, which was masked, is anger originally based on a situation of powerlessness, vis-a-vis her original parents. To break up the Game, another person can simply respond from his Adult which does not automatically accept the *I am a powerless child* secret bait, e.g., *Oh, really? What have you tried?*, and if it becomes clear that *it* will not give up the Game and acknowledge her Adult power to find her own solutions, the other adult can either confront her with her Game or move on to more interesting topics of conversation.

Victims, Persecutors, and Rescuers

Game participants have three positions to play from: *Victim*, *Persecutor*, or *Rescuer*. In the course of the Game these get switched, e.g., in "Why Don't You Yes But" the initiator originally starts as a helpless Victim of the terrible problem and invites someone to be Rescuer. As the Game ends it becomes apparent that he has been persecuting the others and they are Victims of the Game.

I differ from most Transactional Analysts in that I view the essence of a *Game* or set of *Games* a person chooses as an inner flirtation with a core life question, a psychological value imposed by the early Injunctions. This always takes the form of an impasse in which both alternatives are equally feared. The Game insures that neither is faced.

For Anna the core Injunction was *Don't Be*. It took the form of a life question, *Am I wanted or not wanted?* In early school she learned to play "Gee Whiz, Professor, You're Wonderful—You're Unusually Perceptive." She successfully masked her differences of thought and feeling from a succession of male mentors, and avoided the possibility of being seen and valued (with the burden of defining her own position) as well as the possibility of being really seen and rejected. Later with her husband and children she played "Harried." She agreed with all their criticism, accepted all their demands, expected herself to function perfectly as a housekeeper, interior decorator, cook, mother, wife, *and* she said yes to everything extra that was asked of her at work, which occasionally justified a complete collapse (when a critical task would not be done and she caused others to be heavily *let down*). The basic motif was *If I do everything for you, surely you'll want me (but you wouldn't want me if you knew how angry I am)*.

Obviously to play a Game you have to find other people who are willing to play their parts for their own purposes. Selecting partners is much like casting for a play, a few rehearsals determine suitability. What follows is much like a theatrical event: a prescribed cast of characters, dialogue, acts and scenes, themes and plots which can move to a dramatic climax and end with a final curtain or, alternatively, can peter on endlessly like a TV soap opera, going nowhere.

Life Script

The *Life Script*, a TA term for a person's ongoing program for his life, dictates where he is going and how he is going to get there. It is a drama he compulsively acts although his awareness of it may be vague. The man who has taken the position that you can't trust women, marries a sequence of women who let him down. He fulfills his prophecy by selecting a girl who has some indicated potential for nontrust, then he pushes her into situations of trial, complains, becomes jealous, and generally makes life miserable so that eventually she proves his point that *you can't trust women* by taking off with someone else. The woman who marries a series of alcoholics is doing the same thing.

The complementary nature of Scripting in marriage selection can again be illustrated by Anna who selected a man who would never really reassure her that she was wanted or clearly reject her. He seemed totally absorbed in his job as executive in an expanding company. He in turn was in an impasse felt most acutely in his work life, whether or not he had the power to make it to the top. Really dealing with either of these alternatives felt catastrophic to him. If he made it to the top, he would have the burden of constantly proving his ability to stay there, the tension of dealing with other men's envy, and the felt danger of their aggressive competition. If he allowed himself to feel that he did not have the ability (power) to get to the top, he would feel depressed, empty, and suicidal. His major parental Injunction had been *Don't make it.* His Child's decision had been *I'll show you even if it kills me.* The Games he played to avoid resolving the impasse were mostly variants of "If It Weren't for You" although he played his own version of "Harried." Just as his wife tended to project and hear her parental Injunctions as now coming from him, so too he tended to project and hear the *Don't make it* message coming from her and used it to build up, justify, and collect angry feelings (covering the true feeling of fear and anxiety) which made a realistic assessment of his ability unlikely.

Redecisions

Treatment involves analyzing ego states, transactions, Games, Injunctions, Decisions, and Scripts. The core, however, involves one thing to get through the impasse, making a Redecision.

If the person recognizes that he made a wrong Decision at some point in his early life then he can change that Decision. He cannot give up his Injunctions until he stops shifting responsibility, until he lets his parents go, recognizing that they were real people suffering their own disappointments and hurts and passing some of them on, which he can now forgive. He can know the Redecisions that have to be made either by doing the Family Sculpture, or by fantasizing where he will be ten years from now if he continues to follow his Script, and where he will be if he makes a different Decision.

Then he can really begin to change, to stop playing Games, to stop maintaining his Rackets, to stop following his Life Script, and to become autonomous. The real success comes when the client carries out his Redecision to enjoy life, to live, when he no longer denies or restricts his autonomy. He uses different language. He says *I* when he means *I* instead of beginning statements with *You* or *One* or *We*. He says *he won't*, when he means *won't* instead of copping out under words like *try*, *can't*, *want*, *should* and the *why-because* rationalizations. He begins to experience the joy of being free and learns there are other more satisfying kinds of strokes for changing that come from his experience of being himself.

Gestalt techniques focus on awareness and self responsibility in the present moment. Fritz Perls found that people blocked their awareness, their experience of the present by ruminating about the past or fantasizing about the future. He observed that people who seemed more alive and free from anxiety were very much in touch with their current experiencing, met each situation flexibily as it arose. Their responses were spontaneous, required little effort yet seemed centered in some way.

Perls decided this centeredness in the present moment could best be explained by the old German notion of *gestalt* or the pattern of figure and ground. The healthy person is in touch with his own needs either as they arise from within (a need to urinate, a feeling of hunger, or sexual tension) or as opportunities develop outside for the satisfaction of longer term interests and capacities for enjoyment, e.g., he relishes the beauty of a garden or of teaching his child a new skill. These needs and longer term interests and capacities for enjoyment affect his perception of the present moment in a distinct way. The emerging need organizes his field of awareness so the opportunities to meet the need stand out, e.g., the hungry man picks up the aroma of food, the sight of food, and is aware of opportunities to eat. These stimuli become the foreground of his interest until he eats and the rest recedes to the background. Now, however, having satisfied his hunger, his perceptions shift in response to whatever next occupies his interest and the food items recede to the background.

Aside from the body needs of hunger, discharge of wastes, and sexual arousal, Perls observed that most people were in meager contact with their experiences, only half awake to reality. In fact, even with the body needs some people do not do so well. A man can eat automatically, not in response to hunger. He may have sex without enjoyment or, alternatively, be out of touch with sexual hunger. He is either unaware of his specific needs or blocked in demanding what he wants. Often he does not know how to ask or is confused about what he really wants. But once he can express his demands, his requests directly and actually mean what he says, he has made the most important step in feeling his own worth.

Perls defined learning as discovering that something is possible. He said it was possible to discover means and ways to grow but we use most of our energies for self-destructive, self-preventing games because we run away from the unpleasant and the painful. Mostly what we are running from is hurt to our vanity. We do not like to look at that nor at when we feel hurt, we also actually feel vindictive and want to hurt the other person.

So we turn our attention to other things. You can either be in touch with the world, in touch with yourself, or in touch with your fantasy life. When fantasies are taken for a real thing, that is insanity. In our fantasy zone are the catastrophic expectations that distort our view of the world and keep us from meeting our needs simply. But there is also a fantasy of who we are, a self concept that gives us no support. On the contrary, we use it to nag, disapprove, and squash much of our genuine self-expression and along with this we look for approval, affection from others that we won't give ourselves.

One source of confusion between our real self and self-concept is that often we think we should feel either/or, that we should feel love or hate, that we are good or bad. We merely have to replace this with both/and to make it clear that the positive or negative depends on a context. This is much like Jungian psychology's emphasis on the identification and integration of opposites necessary to become an individual.

Gestalt does not provide long explanations of *why* we are as we are. There are no scapegoats to blame. Like giving up the TA Game of "Wooden Leg," we can no longer say *How can you expect me to be any different when I had such a rotten childhood?* Instead, Gestalt has one prescription: Take responsibility; experience yourself as the doer of your actions; stop avoiding, covering up your experience; experience *you*.

Only through integrated spontaniety and deliberateness can we make sound choices. Awareness of our responsibility for the whole field, for the self as well as the other, gives meaning and pattern to our individual life.

Techniques to Stop Avoiding

There are two types of techniques that bring more direct contact with present experiences: One to stop avoiding and the other to intensify attention or exaggerate the experience. These techniques involve stopping the activities that keep us so busy we hardly have any attention left for the moment we are living. There is little place for the *now* in ordinary conversation. We tell stories, share opinions and plans. Even our private mental activity is mostly anticipations, memories, fantasies, and fitting games. Many of these activities emerge in our art experiences indicating how they pervade all aspects of living.

Aboutism. This is what Perls used to call the "Science" Game. He considered the *whys* and *because* of talk most often as rationalization, sheer verbiage, and unsubstantial when weighed against direct experience. Tabooing this type of intellectualizing serves to bring to light what lies hidden behind it, often a sense of emptiness and impotence. Staying with the emptiness, minor feelings begin to evolve like sparks growing into fires. In art experiences of facing the empty sheet of paper until something grows inside that impels expression, it is possible to contact this inner emptiness without words.

Shouldism. Telling ourselves or others what should be is another way of not experienceing what *is*. Evaluating means fitting this now experience to our preestablished standards. We attend to what is missing rather than what is present and often create the unpleasant feelings of frustration rather than awareness of what there is to grasp. In giving up *should*, we stop self-blaming and self-praising. The sign, means, and goal are determined when we can simply acknowledge experience with-out justifying or criticising. In each art exercise, the person's unique expression of his experience is what it is. There is no way it could be *better*.

If we look carefully, we find feelings such as anxiety, guilt, and shame are not direct experiences but the outcome of a mental process. Behind every guilt is the ideal into which we are failing to fit (I should have done a better job; I should be Picasso not me); behind every anxiety, the desire to manipulate the future as we think it should be (You should admire how clever I am).

A goal is a target, a landmark for our orientation, which may be an ideal or not. Gestalt does not seek to eliminate conception of the desirable. It tries to counter an excess of future orientation with good anchorage in the present. *Shoulds* on the other hand oppose a reality that cannot be other than what it is. When we blame ourselves for something past, we do not change the wrongness we concurred in nor is this blaming necessary to do better in the future. Similarly our experiences here and now are what they are; self-blame and self-praise do not change them.

A realistic appraisal of where we are in terms of our aims and ideals is only possible when our evaluation is not biased by the self-punishing game or counteractive defenses. The self-putdown into which we put so much of our energy is altogether different from the serene perception of our failings. The sane attitude towards our failings is similar to that of a good teacher or coach. "That was too high," a tennis coach will say, "Pay attention to your footwork; relax your shoulder more." This takes for granted that you want to use these observations and is very different from demand, manipulation, or control.

Gestalt therapy calls *top-dog* what TA identifies as the Parent ego state. Neither implies that the state should be done away with, only that the state is usually experienced as an imposition of one part of the personality on another. The opposite role is the *underdog* for Gestalt, the Child for TA. Their opposition, whether experienced as an internal battle or whether we manage to induce another person to play one of the opposites, keeps us stuck. The solution in TA and Gestalt is the same as it is in the Jungian approach. We have to identify both aspects as belonging to us. When the opposites are identified, it is possible to assimilate them. *I want* and *I choose* can replace *I should.* The art exercises to identify the opposites of the way we usually think and feel are designed to clarify this inner opposition and make choice possible.

Manipulation

Just as *aboutism* is a misuse of the intellect and *shouldism* is a misuse of the emotions, *manipulation* is a misuse in the sphere of action. For most people, most actions are to avoid a sense of emptiness. One common form of manipulation is to ask questions. Questions not only mask the experience of the questioner but also serve to *suck in* the other to answer and satisfy the questioner's manipulative need. They deviate the content of group interaction away from what is useful. The Gestaltist says, "Make your question into a statement."

Asking for permission is a similar device. Here the individual manipulates the situation so the other takes responsibility for his action and thus the manipulator avoids an impasse, the polarity of his freedom and the fear he feels associated with it. In art therapy all comments by any member of the group on another's work are made using the first person, present tense, and active voice to encourage the members to own their projections and to be responsible for them, and the personal questions they raise.

Expressive and Exaggeration Techniques

In suppressing the cliches, conditioned responses, and games, we become aware of what we are behind these automatic reactions. Exaggerating the expression of impulses heightens awareness of self. Translating your feeling and understanding into words, actions, and forms in art media focuses this sense of aliveness. Expression of a thought, image, or feeling allows an integration of that which was disowned, disassociated from awareness, and therefore ineffective.

The Gestaltist pays close attention to language. He does not allow disowning words, like *it, you,* or *we* when the person means *I*. He doesn't accept *can't* when *won't* is meant. *But* is all too often used to disqualify a statement or to take away some of its force: *Yes, but...; I like you, but...; I'd like to do this but...* In this ambiguity, the individual avoids fully experiencing either half of his statement and each invalidates the other. The Gestaltist then suggests instead using *and. I like you AND I'm annoyed by your timidity* allows a stronger encounter.

The individual is confronted with his own choices to the extent a situation is unstructured. Whatever he does, *he* does.

He chooses to follow or not to follow the dictates of his impulses, wishes, leanings of the moment. The function of the Gestaltist is to make him aware of his own decisions, i.e., he is responsible.

Patient: I am holding my jaw very tight. I feel like screaming.

Therapist: And that you are *not* doing.

Patient: I am afraid it would be ridiculous.

Therapist: It?

Patient: I would feel ridiculous doing such a thing.

Therapist: So here you are in conflict—to scream or to fear the group's opinion.

The conflicts most often manifested are between human needs on the one hand and social roles of behavior and consideration of other people's reactions on the other. Smearing paint and working with clay often evoke impulses unacceptable to the present day adult. Articulating them reopens issues of choice.

Sometimes when the Gestaltist wishes to stimulate initiative and risk-taking, he will suggest *gibberish*, unstructured vocalization. It implies a willingness to say the unknown, the unthought. In its lack of structure there is something that molds itself to our inner reality. Sometimes the person may censor all anger from his words, voice, and awareness and yet produce gibberish that is angry beyond a doubt. When a husband and wife are interacting with gibberish, a range of feelings, pleading, arrogance, may be easily apparent that forms a basic substratum to their relationship. Similarly questions and use of control, power, and initiative are obvious in the unstructured use of paint in a dialogue painting between two people.

Reversal

Reversal assumes that the opposite to what is consciously expressed is also likely to be a part of the person, but a less developed side—attitudes, feelings, physical posture in art, the minor aspect of a painting—when reversed and allowed expression, unfolds unsuspected possibilities and experiences. This is very closely allied again to the Jungian notion of identification and assimilation of the opposites within the personality. When the minister's wife identified with her collage of Raquel Welch as the Roller Derby Queen, this was a reversal which allowed unexpected responses.

One particular type of reversal which Perls emphasized had to do with *retroflection*. This is behavior by which a person does to himself what he originally did or tried to do to other persons or objects. He substitutes himself as the target now because he earlier learned that he could not express those impulses outwardly. He actively holds them back, even from his own awareness, but they get a partial discharge in being turned inward. This is somewhat akin to the TA notion of Rackets which are used to elicit familiar bad feelings but cover up an inner feeling which if owned and allowed discharge would finish the situation. The content varies from person to person. Self-hate, self-pity, self-control, even introspection, Perls considered retroflective peering at oneself and different from genuine self-awareness because observer is split off from the part observed.

In undoing this, the person is asked to translate his self-accusations and guilt into resentment statements, his feelings of being ridiculed into sarcasm directed outward, his feeling of having no right to exist into the hate and anger that lies within. This often can be enacted in psychodrama or mime movement before it can be worded as such.

Finishing situations refers to a person's sense of not completing an act. Words unsaid and things undone leave a trace, binding us to the past. Sometimes this involves a psychodrama, acting a fantasy out, finishing an unfinished dream, saying to parents what was not said to them in childhood, saying goodbye to a divorced spouse or dead relative. What was unsaid, withheld, may have been appreciation or resentment.

A similar phenomenon involves *completing expression.* Nonverbal gesture, tears, and sounds can be translated by giving them a voice. First the gesture is exaggerated, made broader or more precise, more intensively expressive of whatever the initial feeling was. It is then translated: "What is your left hand saying as it squeezes your arm? If your tears could speak, what would they say?" In making the content more explicit, the person contacts his message for himself from the inside. Similarly with the images of a dream or a painting or clay sculpture. In acting them out and giving them voice, we *know* more because being something or someone deepens awareness far more than reasoning about it or him.

These little playlets, or skits as Perls called them, form a major way of owning that which was disassociated and projected, and healing the inner splits within the personality. They bring about the end goal of Gestalt: awareness and self-responsibility in the here and now.

If present-centered here and now awareness is the essence of Gestalt psychology, the catch phrase for depth psychology might be: the beginning of self-knowledge is discovery that I am not only that which I identify myself as being but also that which I strenuously reject (plus much more). The accompanying diagram *THE WHOLE PERSON* pictures the relationship between my conscious mind and the rest of what I am.

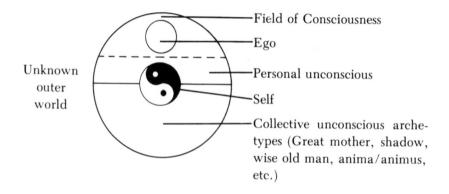

Field of Consciousness

Ego

Unknown outer world

Personal unconscious

Self

Collective unconscious archetypes (Great mother, shadow, wise old man, anima/animus, etc.)

The *Ego* is the small circle floating in its field of consciousness in the upper portion of the diagram. Ego is what I experience as *me* and think of as *I*, the part that wills and chooses. The surrounding field is everything that I am aware of—my friends, people that I dislike, neutral bits of knowledge like mathematics, everything I know. What I am not aware of is either outside the large circle (the unknown outer world) or inside, under my consciousness (the unknown inner world).

This diagram shows that conscious awareness of a friend or of a fact is part of all that I am and is different from your consciousness of that same friend or fact. This fits easily with the Gestalt notion that we each perceive selectively in terms of our needs.

The Task

Jung's chapter "Confrontation with the Unconscious" in his autobiography, *Memories, Dreams, Reflections,* describes how in his own life he used his hands to give form and shape to his unconscious reactions and images. Reproductions of some of his carvings and paintings are found in *C. G. Jung: Word and Image* (Jaffé).

Our task is to bring consciousness and the unconscious into an active and creative relationship. A key to understanding Jung's process of working with the unconscious is found in his essay "The Transcendent Function." In that essay he describes the nature of consciousness and the unconscious:

> (1) Consciousness possesses a threshold intensity which its contents must have attained, so that all elements that are too weak remain in the unconscious.
> (2) Consciousness, because of its directed functions, exercises an inhibition (which Freud calls censorship) on all incompatible material, with the result that it sinks into the unconscious.
> (3) Consciousness constitutes the momentary process of adaptation, whereas the unconscious contains not only all the forgotten material of the individual's own past, but all the inherited behavior traces constituting the structure of the mind.
> (4) The unconscious contains all the fantasy combinations which have not yet attained the threshold intensity, but which in the course of time and under suitable conditions will enter the light of consciousness. (*CW*, vol. 8, p. 69)

The publisher gratefully acknowledges the use of excerpts from *The Collected Works of C. G. Jung* (hereinafter referred to as *CW*), trans. R. F. C. Hull, Bollingen Series XX, Vol. 8: *The Structure and Dynamics of the Psyche,* copyright © 1960, 1969 by Princeton University Press, pp. 69, 70–71, 86–87, and 88–89, and Vol. 9, II: *Aion: Researches into the Phenomenology of the Self,* copyright © 1959 by Princeton University Press, p. 5. The excerpts are reprinted by permission of Princeton University Press. The publisher is also grateful to Routledge & Kegan Paul Ltd. (London), publisher of the above-mentioned edition of *The Collected Works of C. G. Jung* in England, for permission to reprint these excerpts.

Consciousness as we know it today, so essential to science, technology, and civilization, developed relatively late in the history of the human race. Since it is important that each individual's conscious awareness be as stable as possible, psychic elements that appear to be incompatible with what is known consciously tend to be inhibited or excluded when we make choices.

> Through such acts of judgment the directed process necessarily becomes one-sided, even though the rational judgment may appear many-sided and unprejudiced. The very rationality of the judgment may even be the worst prejudice, since we call reasonable what appears reasonable to us. What appears to us unreasonable is therefore doomed to be excluded because of its irrational character. It may really be irrational, but may equally well merely appear irrational without actually being so when seen from another standpoint. (CW, vol. 8, pp. 70–71)

The further we remove ourselves from the unconscious, the more likely it is that a strong counterposition can build up, which will have disagreeable consequences when it breaks out. What kind of mental and moral attitude can we take toward these disturbing influences in the unconscious? What is this task we are defining? Somehow we have to recognize the significance of the unconscious in compensating the one-sidedness of consciousness. We must relate to both the conscious and the unconscious data in order to arrive at a new, transcendent attitude.

Dreams and unconscious interferences in the waking state—slips of the tongue, for example—point to the missing or compensating unconscious contents that we need to pay attention to. Most signals from the unconscious lack sufficient continuity for a meaningful synthesis with consciousness; however, a capacity to produce sustained free fantasies *can* be developed. For example, one can use an uncomfortable emotional state such as a depression or an irritable mood to stimulate objective exploration by sinking into such a state without reserve and noting all the fantasies and associations that come up. A picture may appear that clarifies the contents and tendencies of the unconscious that were massed together. This is the beginning of what Jung called the transcendent function, i.e., using both conscious and unconscious data in shaping symbolic images that could not be achieved by consciousness alone.

One way of dealing with emotional disturbance, i.e., this push of the unconscious, is to give it visible shape in a drawing or painting. It is important not for the picture to be technically satisfying or artistic but for the fantasy to have free play. For some people, this can take the form of inner dialogue. Others neither see nor hear anything inside themselves, but their hands seem to know how to release meaning and form in clay or other materials. The family sculpture is a creative example of the hands "knowing."

> The unconscious contents want first of all to be seen clearly, which can only be done by giving them shape, and to be judged only when everything they have to say is tangibly present. . . .
> . . . The kind of understanding with which we are concerned at this stage consists in a reconstruction of the meaning that seems to be immanent in the original "chance" idea. (*CW*, vol. 8, pp. 86–87)

Once the unconscious contents have been given form, how should the ego relate to it? At this point, the unconscious no longer takes the lead; it is now up to the ego—that continuous center of choice-making and consciousness.

The task has difficulties that Jung described:

> There is a danger of the ego losing its head, so to speak, that it will not be able to defend itself against the pressure of affective factors—a situation often encountered at the beginning of schizophrenia. This danger would not exist, or would not be so acute, if the process of having it out with the unconscious could somehow divest the affects of their dynamism. And this is what does in fact happen when the counter-position is aestheticized or intellectualized. But the confrontation with the unconscious must be a many-sided one, for the transcendent function is not a partial process running a conditioned course; it is a total and integral event in which all aspects are,

or should be, included. The affect must therefore be deployed in its full strength. Aestheticization and in-tellectualization are excellent weapons against dan-gerous affects, but they should be used only when there is a vital threat, and *not for the purpose of avoiding a necessary task.* . . .

. . . the treatment of neurosis is not a kind of psychological water-cure, but a renewal of the per-sonality, working in every direction and penetrating every sphere of life. Coming to terms with the counter-position is a serious matter on which some-times a very great deal depends. Taking the other side seriously is an essential prerequisite of the pro-cess, for only in that way can the regulating factors exert an influence on our actions. Taking it seriously does not mean taking it literally, but it does mean giving the unconscious credit, so that it has a chance to co-operate with consciousness instead of automat-ically disturbing it. . . .

The present day shows with appalling clarity how little able people are to let the other man's ar-gument count, although this capacity is a fundamen-tal and indispensable condition for any human com-munity. Everyone who proposes to come to terms with himself must reckon with this basic problem. For, to the degree that he does not admit the validity of the other person, he denies the "other" within himself the right to exist—and vice versa. The capac-ity for inner dialogue is a touchstone for outer objec-tivity. (Italics added; *CW*, vol. 8, pp. 88–89)

Functions of Art Methods in Therapy

The psychotherapist using these insights from Jung will facili-tate his patient's widening of consciousness during an emotional crisis not only with words but also through encouraging the pa-tient to give some tangible shape to inner images.

Using art materials to make images and connecting them to feelings and body states brings into the open emotions and thoughts that have been only vaguely sensed. Closure becomes possible for unfinished issues that push for resolution—for ex-ample, in reconnection to unfinished or blocked feelings of the loss-grieving cycle.

People often come to therapy in a state of depression connected with death, divorce, loss of a parent, a lover, or a child, loss of role, or loss of self-esteem through failure to make a scholastic or professional goal. Any one of these can set in motion a sequence of reactions similar to the grieving cycle and can be treated as such. The sequence is never as uncomplicated as shown in the following figure, but the art processes sometimes indicate possibilities for reorganization. They can deepen the emotional experience and elicit behavioral responses that may have been blocked.

LOSS-GRIEVING CYCLE

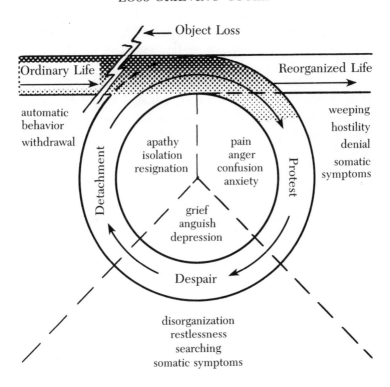

Note: Based on the sequence outlined by John Bowlby, M.D., and developed by William M. Lamers, Jr., M.D.; also described in Margaret Keyes, "The Mobilization of Affect in Women Through Art," in *Emotional Flooding*, New Directions in Psychotherapy, vol. 1, ed. P. Olsen (New York: Human Sciences, 1976), pp. 151–76.

Following loss there are commonly three periods of reaction: protest, despair, and detachment. After detachment, a period of reorganization of one's life begins. Inside the circle of the diagram are the emotions experienced within the person; outside the circle are the behavioral counterparts that others observe. During the phase of protest, tears serve as a sign of distress and a call for help. Hostility expresses anger directed two ways: at the object (the lover, parents, child) for going away and, in a sense, as a warning never to go away again; and at the self for having caused the rupture. Denial allows the belief that what the senses say has happened has not. Memory disturbances function in the same way. Somatic symptoms—sighing, muscular weakness, disturbed sleep, and diminished appetite—indicate the self's need and dependence. Despair is outwardly manifested in disorganization, restlessness, and searching. Inwardly there is anguish and depression. During detachment, emotional affect tends to flatten to apathy and resignation. Outer behavior is automatic with a tendency to withdraw from personal relationships. If the loss can be integrated and new relationships formed, personality reorganization and reintegration take place.

Once one has worked out these issues, it is then possible to get out of the repetitive cycles and to move onto the reorganization track. Table 1, relating art processes to the phases of the loss cycle, is intended simply to suggest possibilities for the design of treatment.

Table 1

ART PROCESSES RELATED TO PHASES
OF LOSS-GRIEVING CYCLE

PHASE	PROCESSES	PURPOSES
Protest	Sculpting relationships	To develop feelings toward parent, mate, child
	Family sculpture	To develop Transactional Analysis injunctions that therapist can use to trigger bioenergetic exercises, Altered States of Consciousness (ASC), and early family scenes to work through and experience feelings that are blocked
	Clay smearing	To release disgust and anger through regression
	Shadow collage	To connect with projected feelings
	Painting body images	To contact and connect body constriction, areas of deadness, evidence of loss or hurt, images of what was and of what is wanted, and yearnings
Despair	Painting feelings	To develop images of inner and outer aspects of loss and of felt conflicts, later used in integration painting, polarization, and dialogue painting; to identify tension within or in relation to partner
	Enacting dream images with psychodrama and videotape	To enter into feelings of blackness and emptiness; to deepen feelings of loss and then say good-bye
Detachment	Use of journal in work with myths and structured dialogues	To identify knowledge gained; to recognize importance of including darkness and possibilities for rebirth; to recognize and contain feelings within images; to connect images to process of transformation

Table 1 (continued)

ART PROCESSES RELATED TO PHASES
OF LOSS-GRIEVING CYCLE

PHASE	PROCESSES	PURPOSES
Reorganization	Painting dream images; mandalas*; collages; visual and audio assemblage of images and music, i.e., "autobiography" of lines of poetry combined with excerpts of music important in various phases of one's life, presented with artifacts, pictures, and photographs from same periods	To stimulate activity and further work of integration and growth; to identify and contain opposite feelings (both/and rather than either/or)
	Painting images from ASC fantasies	To further analogous thought of options and possibilities

*These are not intended to represent the spontaneous healing symbols that emerge in the process of individuation; rather, they are meditation drawings.

This type of psychotherapy using the arts characteristically releases a significant amount of energy. The blocked negative feelings have been recovered and have to be experienced before reorganization can occur. Conscious love has to encounter unconscious resentment before forgiveness, empathy, and true caring can be achieved. So, too, conscious resentment has to encounter unconscious love.

In the process of living one's life it is necessary to experience one's opposed inner urges to allow a transcendent synthesis. Table 2 indicates some points in the life cycle when such oppositions constellate.

The issues in table 2 may occur in different decades or in different sequences from those outlined—and certainly no one experiences all of them—but these are critical points for many people and, as such, any one of them can bring on an encounter between consciousness and the unconscious.

In using art methods and active imagination to understand these periods of transition, we find that the symbol-images that arise spontaneously are the best possible way to represent meanings as yet unknown or difficult to grasp. The symbol-images are frequently metaphors for our daily struggles, fears, and preoccupations. Reflecting on them can move one to an awareness of the many moments when images are lived in one's life. In responding to the images, one experiences spontaneous transformations in behavior and understanding. Sometimes the images work out their own solutions.

Table 2

CONTEMPORARY PROBLEM AREAS AND ISSUES IN LIFE CYCLE

PASSING FROM CHILDHOOD TO ADULTHOOD

Teens	Sexual activity: self-esteem, peer pressure, emotional readiness, lack of awareness (despite sex education) of different meaning of sex to men and to women, personal realization of effects of pregnancy and abortion
	Involvement of parents (in late thirties and forties) in unresolved issues of value and self-esteem
	Pop culture: false consciousness; illusions about self, society, political order, life; media focus on commercial values that trivializes, homogenizes, stereotypes people, manipulates and debases sex, oversimplifies life
	Competition, idealism, cults, mind-altering substances and situations: oversimple answers that substitute for tasks of consciousness
Twenties	Love affairs: damage to self-esteem from multiple affairs, loss, premature closure, leading to closing off emotionally and sexually, to substitution of relations with same sex, to confusion about anger and rights versus relatedness
	Career: how much energy to invest; how to act when one perceives that career doesn't meet ideal standards—e.g., when young lawyer realizes that many aspects of law are not concerned with justice
	Spiritual values: live-now materialism versus idealism

MARRYING, CHILDBEARING, AND/OR INVESTING IN CAREER

Thirties	Need for work or professional training to be recognized; in profession, development of power and influence
	Need for cultivated intimacy; need for sense of meaningful direction
	For women, confusion about allocation of energy and work style. For single women, pregnancy in or out of marriage, relationships with married men, marriage to divorced man who does not want another child, anger at potential mate's

Table 2 (continued)

CONTEMPORARY PROBLEM AREAS AND ISSUES IN LIFE CYCLE

	immaturity, materialism, lack of commitment. For married women, lack of communication with husband, few common interests with him, money problems connected to inflation and overextended debt, need for separate time or day off to study or cultivate interests, balance of time between profession and marriage (work versus home)
Forties	Because of children in teens, reactivation of questions about self-esteem and value of work, marriage, career; meaningful midlife transitions
	With late children, special out-of-phase problems
	Six addictions (food, drugs, alcohol, work, gambling, and TV) that divert energy and repress consciousness

ENDINGS AND SHIFTINGS IN MARRIAGE, WORK, AND BODY

Fifties	Decision-making adjustments, e.g., when wife wants voice in questions of refinancing home or using her separate property to promote husband's business ventures
	Extramarital affairs (typically husband with younger businesswoman or wife with old friend); sexual incompatibility
	Career uncertainty, strong investment in new life direction, "empty nest" syndrome, home-based enriched and cultivated life (including community service)
	For women, menopause: physical symptoms, attractiveness, self-worth, being wanted and needed, increasing awareness of spiritual values and outer-world issues
Sixties	Economic issues and loss of self-esteem related to decrease in income
	Infirmity and death of parents; own aging; serious illness of friends
	Spiritual issues
	Retirement: sharing space and increased time with spouse

AGING AND DYING

Seventies	Sensory impairment: outer endings and inward focus
	Ability to live with pain
	Integration of view of own life
Eighties	Family relationships
	Ability to make own decisions

Life crises are times when we are forced to deal with opposing desires or points of view that become embodied in these images. Often the images suggest that certain traits and habit patterns are organized around specific drives or urges that are in conflict. A single parent may find her mothering aspect dominant at the cost of her sexual woman or the reverse. From a metaphorical point of view, these images can be described as sub-personalities—and in a certain sense the sub-personalities can be thought of as the archetypes in contemporary dress (as shown in the figure on the next page.)

Sub-personalities (or "complexes") are developed from a pool of human traits that we all share. The particular form is often based on an early family experience unconsciously preserved, e.g., a "father's girl" behaves differently from a "mother's girl," and so the "eternal girl" archetype is therefore more or less available to a given individual. Introjects from parents, teachers, and therapists can also form the ground of a sub-personality and provide a channel for archetypal imagery.

Charting sub-personalities at a time of crisis can be a highly useful exercise. One can use the spontaneously developed images and also customary roles (physician, mother, church member, daughter, PTA secretary) to investigate how one experiences oneself and what others observe in physical appearance, dress, or positive and negative emotional states. Language and style of speech often change as one changes roles, and certain phrases are typical. One notes also which situations or emotional attitudes trigger a change in role.

ARCHETYPES, SUB-PERSONALITIES, AND LIFE CYCLE

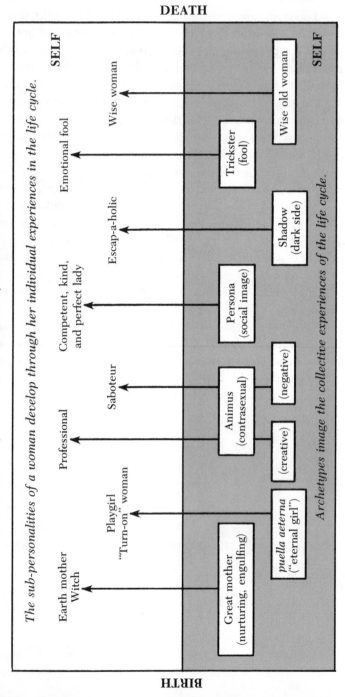

The sub-personalities of a woman develop through her individual experiences in the life cycle.

Archetypes image the collective experiences of the life cycle.

Tables 3 and 4 develop the sub-personalities of one woman and one man as examples of this work of transformation of inner conflicting elements. For Molly, a crisis began when her only son was killed in a car accident. The lack of any emotional bond in her marriage apart from the adolescent son was then apparent. Assembling the table made clear to her that her "Turn-On" persona, active in initiating the marriage, had not developed a capacity for intimacy. This function was carried by the Believer (a mother's daughter), whose characteristics were particularly difficult for her husband to see and value. This in turn activated the Saboteur in her and a Mafia Con Man shadow aspect in her husband. Understanding her own inner needs better, Molly was able to relax her professional drive, which had served to distract her from the painful lack of fulfillment in any other area of her life. The Saboteur and Escap-a-holic then largely disappeared, and her long-suppressed artistic ability began to surface.

In Clyde's situation, not only his marriage but his business life was in trouble. He needed a better relationship with his own feeling side, and he constantly sought this in extramarital sexual relations. Unacknowledged feelings were also at the root of his work difficulties. He was competing with his father's successful business in the same field. He overlooked the fact that his father had taken years to build his success. Clyde demanded of himself that he surpass anything that his father accomplished. Proving to the old man that he did not need him, Clyde overlooked how much he still wanted his father's love and approval. Neither father nor son was comfortable with tender feelings. It took a couple of years of psychotherapy before Clyde could finally acknowledge this, but then he no longer had to invest his total being in his work drive as he reclaimed more of his range of feelings. For both Clyde and Molly, charting the sub-personalities provided a starting place for active-imagination dialogue and journal work.

When one lives unconsciously, i.e., when one's ego identifies more or less totally with a favorite role or way of being in the world, awareness tends to be limited to the perceptions screened by that mind set. There is often a sense of personal powerlessness but paradoxically an inclination to manipulate others to do one's will and take a similar point of view. An al-

Table 3
SUB-PERSONALITIES OF MOLLY

Sub-Personality (Complex)	Functional Types	Roles	Attributes (Physical + Emotional + Mental + Spiritual)	Language Phrases	Origins	Triggers
"Turn-on" woman (persona)	Extrovert Feeling Sensation	Hostess Homemaker Teacher Workshop leader	Physically attractive, enjoys vivid clothes and unique jewelry, high energy, colorful, infectious enthusiasm, earthly, slightly salty tongue, humor, bright, responsive, connects people with one another, individualizes *Wants*: Admiration, interplay, excitement with interesting people, but not intimacy or equality *Needs*: People to care about and interact with in varied ways, to be given to, to have egocentric self-sufficiency broken	"All work and no play" is turning me into a nerd.	"Show-biz" grand-mother Family okay on massage and body care	Small groups of her public Attractive men
Escap-a-holic (shadow)	Introvert Intuitive Feeling	Failure	Physically unattractive, lonely, hopeless beyond self-pity, mentally turned off, passive, spiritually desperate, eats too much, drinks too much, watches TV addictively, work-a-holic *Wants*: To be taken care of; to escape from responsibilities, pain, aloneness, emptiness, sense of having failed to love *Needs*: To be loved for what she is, not what she can do	Nothing matters because I matter to no one.	Conditional love from parents Childhood of escape routes into books linked to work-a-holic escape into other people's lives	Situation where unseen or unvalued
Artist	Introvert Feeling Intuition and sensation balanced	Seer Dancer Craftsman	Physically aware, particularly of textures; loses self in writing, sculpting, seeing pattern and form; not interested in doing for others but delights in products; "selfish"; feels exploited and used by Professional sub-personality; resents lack of time to develop skill; noncompetitive *Wants*: Time and opportunity *Needs*: Time and opportunity	See and celebrate.	Father who wrote and painted	Access to good material and creative people Experiences in art school

Table 3 (continued)

SUB-PERSONALITIES OF MOLLY

Professional (creative animus)	Extrovert Intuitive Thinking	Lawyer Teacher Writer	Indifferent to physical appearance, projects high energy, enthusiasm, quick here-now intelligence, aware but impersonally involved, detached, highly principled, visionary, fascinated by interrelationship of ideas, effective in packaging and selling ideas, self-advertising, commercial, competent, very hard working, dominating *Wants:* Power, acclaim, precision, effectiveness *Needs:* Appropriate sphere and limitation of territorial ambitions	Life is serious. Work is all that matters. Look, it's obvious. Let me diagram it.	Surgeon father Unfulfilled ambitions and anger of mother	Almost anything
Believer (daughter of great mother)	Introvert Intuitive Feeling	Wife Mother Contributor to altruistic causes One who has private religious experiences Writer and teacher of ethics	Indifferent to physical appearance; accepts poverty values related to social injustice; sad, grieving, doubtful, uncertain, frightened; caring; feels tears frequently close to surface; slow thinker; mystic visionary; accepts death, failure, rebirth sequences in life; accepts searching for wisdom and meaning; passive, low energy; passionately cares about individual friendships but also has Emily Dickinson–quality of inner arrogance *Wants:* Time to worship, express, and explore *Needs:* Worship-prayer life, time to connect insights from other sub-personalities	My purpose in life is to know, to love, and to serve.	Mother's religious values Religious schooling including graduate studies Early nature experiences in Sierra Elitist readings and friendships	Early morning solitude Friend's letters
Saboteur (negative animus)	Extrovert Sensation Thinking	Wife	Physically unattractive, feels poor, will not attend to health and beauty concerns, suspicious, defiant, feels powerless, picky, constricted consciousness, tight throat, bigoted, narrow, whiny, challenging, indirectly attacking, slippery justifier *Wants:* Revenge, recognition *Needs:* To be given to, to have underlying values accepted	You don't appreciate me. I'll show you. Who needs you?	Relation with father	Criticism or feeling unseen

Table 4

SUB-PERSONALITIES OF CLYDE

SUB-PERSONALITY (COMPLEX)	FUNCTIONAL TYPES	ROLES	ATTRIBUTES (PHYSICAL + EMOTIONAL + MENTAL + SPIRITUAL)	LANGUAGE PHRASES	ORIGINS	TRIGGERS
Competitor (persona)	Extrovert Thinking	Executive Mountain climber	Soft voice, diffident manner, hypertense, works hard, plays hard, competent, gambles high in calculated risks *Wants:* First place *Needs:* Territory	Be the best!	Introject of father's persona	Opportunity of almost any kind
Perfectionist engineer	Introvert Sensation	Businessman Socializer Musician	Aware of details to point of nitpicking but can work with large number of variables, machinelike, indifferent to feeling, frightened of being trapped *Wants:* Praise *Needs:* Caring	Be perfect or don't do it. Don't embarrass (me).	Child's relation with mother	Unwanted emotions
Sadist (shadow)	Extrovert Feeling	Businessman Highway driver	Vengeful, arrogant, contemptuous, likes to play with people's emotions, feels omnipotent, takes high risks that go beyond reason *Wants:* Revenge *Needs:* Justice	He's not acting according to *my* rules, and I'm going to get him.	Mother's negative animus	Frustration, opposition, "the smell of blood"
Feeling one (anima)	Introvert Feeling	Husband Father Socializer Musician	Tearful; sadness wells up unexpectedly; inarticulate; ability to write poetry and to paint and draw stifled by perfectionist; capacity for relationship, caring, comforting, and self-sacrifice *Wants:* To be allowed out *Needs:* Love and friendship	(wordless)	Hidden childhood	Awareness of vulnerability in woman, beauty in situation, unmet need for caring
Casanova lover (*puer aeternus*)	Extrovert Sensation	Boss	"Calm and relaxed"; likes to please women, lots of them, and to be acknowledged as the best; won't be captured; cuts out when feeling threatens *Wants:* Power, recognition *Needs:* Relationship	Have fun, but don't get too involved. I'm the greatest.	Relation with mother	Whatever game (heterosexual) is offered

coholic mother said she had never made a real choice until she decided on sobriety. She had drifted into a teaching job, then marriage and having children. When she was sober, she said she finally could let her children have their own lives instead of manipulating them. She could accept her husband's choices as different from hers instead of acting as if she were his victim.

As one differentiates one's choices from collective patterns, the self, a totality and unity of inner opposites, becomes manifest. As one successfully deals with opposing desires or points of view within oneself, one's identity shifts from the ego to a deeper, more objective center of one's being, the self, which includes the total personality. "The ego is, by definition, subordinate to the self and is related to it like a part to the whole" (*CW*, vol. 9, part II, p. 5).

The state of mind that results from a cycle of work like that described by Molly and Clyde is concerned with *being* more than *doing;* it is concerned with a quality of "awakeness" rather than a quantity of accomplishments and experiences. It is not, however, an esoteric or aesthetic state of consciousness, for a practical here-and-now involvement and concern with the everyday world is equally characteristic.

The need to find and to accept inner aspects of oneself is almost a mini-model of what is needed in the outer world. There we have the problem of how to relate to people who do not share our beliefs and attitudes, whose power interests are different from our own. Whether we come to terms with this as our task or whether we keep trying to play "we're right, you're wrong" games with our enemies is the question in the outer world as in our inner experience. How do we change our conflicts to authentic dialogues? The difficulty is undeniable, but possibly by identifying who our "inner revolutionaries" and our "inner Soviets" are and by hearing what those rejected parts want as well as what the official us wants, we can learn to engage in real dialogues. We can then contribute more fully to the collective consciousness of humankind.

Bibliography

Adler, G. 1961. *The living symbol.* New York: Pantheon.

————. 1979. *Dynamics of the self.* London: Coventure.

Anderson, M., and L. Savary. 1971. *Passages: A guide for pilgrims of the mind.* New York: Harper and Row.

This beautifully designed book introduces the beginner to the techniques of relaxation and trance induction for specific purposes: to enhance creativity, to change one's weight or body functioning, and so on.

Arnheim, R. 1982. *Art and visual perception: A psychology of the creative eye, the new version.* Berkeley, Calif.: University of California Press.

Bach, S. 1980. Spontaneous images at critical moments of life: A contribution of the relation between psyche and soma. *Psychosomatische medizin.* Solothurn, Switz.: Hans Huber. (Articles are in English.)

Baker, I. F., ed. 1980. *Methods of treatment in analytical psychology.* VIIth International Congress of the International Association for Analytical Psychology. Stuttgart: Verlag Adolf Bonz. Distributed in the United States by Spring Publications, Dallas.

Benton, S. 1975. *The art of welded sculpture.* New York: Van Nostrand Reinhold.

Berensohn, P. 1968. *Finding one's way with clay.* New York: Simon and Schuster.

Berensohn teaches a unique application of human imagination to clay and water. This is a craftsman's journal of observation and practice in his search for artistic and spiritual growth.

Berger, J. 1978. *Ways of seeing.* London: Penguin Books.

The way we see things is affected by what we know or what we believe. An image is interpreted in its context. Images in a consumer society are used to interpret the world in a starkly different way from its actual condition and to impose a false (and unconscious) standard of what is and is not desirable. Berger uses series of images to make his points nonverbally as well as in text.

————. 1980. *About looking.* New York: Random House.

By examining animals in the wild and animals in zoos, then photographing them ("The most mysterious of all objects that make up and thicken the environment we recognize as modern"), Berger awakens our awareness of the functional use of images. This profound and thoughtful book explores our experience of meaning and meaninglessness.

Berne, E. 1961. *Transactional analysis in psychotherapy.* New York: Grove Press.

————. 1963. *The structure and dynamics of organizations and groups.* New York: Grove Press.

————. 1972. *What do you say after you say hello?* New York: Grove Press.

Birkhauser, P. 1980. *Light from the darkness, the paintings of Peter Birkhauser.* Basel, Switz.: Birkhauser Verlag.

Bolander, K. 1977. *Assessing personality through tree drawings.* New York: Basic Books.

Bonney, H., and L. Savary. 1973. *Music and your mind: Listening with a new consciousness*. San Francisco: Harper & Row.
The techniques of body relaxation and active imagination using music to facilitate mood exploration are described, with specific classical-music referents.

Campbell, J. 1974. *The mythic image*. Princeton: Princeton University Press.

Castillejo, I. C. de. 1973. *Knowing woman*. New York: Harper Colophon Books.

Cirlot, J. E. *A dictionary of symbols*. New York: Philosophical Library.

Cook, R. 1974. *The tree of life: Symbol of the centre*. Art and Imagination Series. London: Thames and Hudson.

Cooper, J. C. 1978. *An illustrated encyclopedia of traditional symbols*. London: Thames and Hudson.

Coudert, J. 1965. *Advice from a failure*. New York: Dell.

Cousins, N. 1981. *Anatomy of an illness*. New York: Bantam.

Coxhead, D., and S. Hiller. N.d. *Dreams: Visions of the night*. Art and Imagination Series. London: Thames and Hudson.

Dallett, J. 1982. The practice of active imagination. In *Jungian analysis*, ed. M. Stein. La Salle, Ill.: Open Court.

Edwards, B. 1979. *Drawing on the right side of the brain*. Los Angeles: J. P. Tarcher.

Fagain, J., and I. L. Shepard. 1970. *Gestalt therapy now*. Palo Alto, Calif.: Science and Behavior Books.

Field, J. 1981. *A life of one's own*. Los Angeles: J. P. Tarcher.
A long-out-of-print classic, this journal reports a true inward journey and describes a method of experiment and close attention to one's consciousness that resulted in the author's discovery that she was not the creature she thought. "For what is really easy, as I found, is to blind one's eyes to what one really likes, to drift into accepting one's wants, ready made from other people, and to evade the continual day-to-day sifting of values." Gradually coming to understand forces that limited her power of perception, the author became aware of an unconscious wisdom wiser than she.

Franz, M.-L. von. 1963. *Interpretation of fairytales, an introduction to the psychology of fairytales*. Dallas: Spring Publications.

———. 1972. *Creation myths*. Zurich: Spring Publications.

———. 1980a. On active imagination. In *Methods of treatment in analytical psychology*, ed. I. F. Baker. Stuttgart: Verlag Adolf Bonz. Distributed in the United States by Spring Publications, Dallas.

———. 1980b. *Projection and re-collection in Jungian psychology: Reflections of the soul*. Translated by William H. Kennedy. La Salle, Ill.: Open Court.

Gardner, H. 1980. *Artful scribbles: The significance of children's drawings*. New York: Harper Colophon Books.

———. 1982. *Art, mind and brain: A cognitive approach to creativity*. New York: Basic Books.

Goulding, M. M., and R. Goulding. 1979. *Changing lives through redecision therapy*. New York: Brunner/Mazel.

Guggenbühl, A. 1971. *Power in the helping professions*. New York: Spring Publications.

Halifax, J. 1979. *Shamanic voices: A survey of visionary narratives*. New York: Dutton.

Hammer, E. F. 1975. *The clinical application of perspective drawings.* Springfield, Ill.: C. C. Thomas.

Hannah, B. 1981. *Encounters with the soul: Active imagination.* Santa Monica, Calif.: Sigo Press.

Harding, M. E. 1970. *The way of all women.* New York: Putnam.

———. 1971. *The "I" and the "Not-I."* Princeton: Princeton University Press.

Hill, G., ed. 1981. *Sandplay studies: Origins, theory and practice.* San Francisco: Jung Institute.

Howes, E., and S. Moon. 1977. *The choice maker.* A Quest Book. Wheaton, Ill.: Theosophical Publishing.

Hull, R. F. C. 1971. Bibliographical notes on active imagination in the works of C. G. Jung. *Spring:* 115–20.

Jacobi, J. 1965. *The way of individuation.* London: Hodder and Stoughton.

Jaffé, A. 1979. *C. G. Jung: Word and image.* Princeton: Princeton University Press.

James, M., and L. Savary. 1977. *A new self: Self therapy with transactional analysis.* Menlo Park, Calif.: Addison-Wesley.

Jung, C. G. 1950– . *The collected works of C. G. Jung.* Ed. R. F. C. Hull. Bollingen Series XX. Princeton: Princeton University Press.

———. 1958. *Psyche and symbols.* Ed. V. de Laszlo. New York: Doubleday.

———. 1960. The transcendent function. In *Collected works,* vol. 8, pp. 67–91. Princeton: Princeton University Press.

———. 1961. *Memories, dreams, reflections.* New York: Random House, Vintage Books.

———. 1964. *Man and his symbols.* Garden City, N.Y.: Doubleday.

Jung, E. 1969. *Animus and anima.* New York: Spring Publications.

Kalff, D. 1980. *Sandplay.* Santa Monica, Calif.: Sigo Press.
    Dora Kalff describes a series of experiences of children using the miniature figures in a sand tray to tell stories and work on their psychological problems through the use of images.

Kellog, R. 1967. *The psychology of children's art.* New York: Random House.

———. 1969. *Analyzing children's art.* Palo Alto, Calif.: Mayfield.

Keyes, M. 1976a. Art processes evoking awareness of the shadow archetype. *Art Psychotherapy* 3 (spring): 77–80.

———. 1976b. The mobilization of affect in women through art. In *Emotional flooding,* New Directions in Psychotherapy, vol. 1, ed. P. Olsen. New York: Human Sciences.

———. 1978. Dante and the tasks of individuation. *Art Psychotherapy* 5 (winter).

Koestler, A. 1964. *The act of creation.* New York: Macmillan.

Kramer, E. 1974. *Art as therapy with children.* New York: Schocken.

———. 1980. *Childhood and art therapy.* New York: Schocken.

Langer, S. K. 1962. *Philosophical sketches.* Baltimore: Johns Hopkins University Press.

Lüscher, M. 1969. *The Lüscher color test.* New York: Simon and Schuster.

Machover, K. A. 1957. *Personality projection in the drawing of the human figure: A method of personality investigation.* Springfield, Ill.: C. C. Thomas.

Maclagan, D. 1979. *Creation myths: Man's introduction to the world.* Art and Imagination Series. London: Thames and Hudson.

Matthews, J. 1981. *The grail: Quest for the eternal.* Art and Imagination Series. New York: Crossroads; London: Thames and Hudson.

Mattoon, M. A. 1982. *Jungian psychology in perspective.* Riverside, N.J.: The Free Press.

Michell, J. 1975. *The earth spirit.* Art and Imagination Series. New York: Crossroads.

Mindell, A. 1982. *Dreambody.* Santa Monica, Calif.: Sigo Press.

Moon, S. 1970. *A magic dwells.* Middletown, Conn.: Wesleyan University Press.

Naranjo, C. 1973. *The techniques of gestalt therapy.* Berkeley, Calif.: SAT Press.

Neumann, E. 1973. *Depth psychology and a new ethic.* New York: Harper Torch Books.

Ornstein, R. 1973. *The psychology of consciousness.* San Francisco: Freeman.

Parenti, M. 1978. *Power and the powerless.* New York: St. Martin's.
This book presents the interface between inner-world and outer-world issues of power and powerlessness.

Perls, F. 1969. *Gestalt therapy verbatim.* Lafayette, Calif.: Real People Press.

_____. 1973. *The gestalt approach.* Palo Alto, Calif.: Science and Behavior Books.

Prinzhorn, H. 1972. *Artistry of the mentally ill.* New York: Springer Verlag.

Purce, J. 1974. *The mystic spiral: Journey of the soul.* Art and Imagination Series. London: Thames and Hudson.

Reed, J. 1975. *Sand magic: Experience in miniature, a non-verbal therapy for children.* Albuquerque, N.M.: JPR press.
A slim volume, quickly read.

_____. 1980. *Emergence: Essays on the process of individuation through sand tray therapy, art forms, and dreams.* Albuquerque, N.M.: JPR Press.
This New Mexican Jungian brings a richly creative American point of view to her methods of therapy. Her groupings and list of sand-tray figures powerfully evoke the possibilities of this medium.

Rhyne, J. 1973. *The gestalt art experience.* Belmont, Calif.: Brooks/Cole.

Richards, M. 1970. *Centering—in pottery, poetry and the person.* Middletown, Conn.: Wesleyan University Press.
An engrossing presentation of the interlinked awareness of psychological issues and growth in the "doing and making" of pottery and poetry.

Robertson, S. 1982. *Rosegarden and labyrinth.* Dallas, Tex.: Spring Publications.
Originally published in 1963, this book is a must for anyone who works with children. It describes the embodiment of the human spirit in children work-playing with art, using materials provided by the teacher-author in different settings. Art as a reflection of the evolving, integrating growth of the child is well illustrated by specific examples, including those in the title.

Rubin, J. 1978. *Child art therapy.* New York: Van Nostrand Reinhold.

Sexton, M. P. 1975. *The Dante-Jung correspondence.* Northridge, Calif.: Joyce Motion Picture.

Stein, M., ed. 1982. *Jungian analysis.* La Salle, Ill.: Open Court.

Steiner, C. M. 1975. *Scripts people live.* New York: Bantam.

Stevens, A. 1982. *Archetypes: A natural history of the self, a pioneering investigation into the biological basis of Jung's theory of archetypes.* New York: William Morrow.

Turner, V. 1967. *Forest of symbols.* Ithaca, N.Y.: Cornell University Press.

Uhlin, D. 1972. *Art for exceptional children.* Dubuque, Iowa: Brown Co.

Ulanov, A. 1971. *The feminine.* Evanston, Ill.: Northwestern University Press.

Ulman, E., ed. *American journal of art therapy.* Washington, D.C.: American Art Therapy Association.

Ulman, E., and C. Levy. 1980. *Art therapy viewpoints.* New York: Schocken.

Virshup, E. 1978. *Right-brain people in a left-brain world.* Los Angeles: Guild of Tutors Press.

Von Ditfurth, H. 1974. *Children of the cosmos.* New York: Atheneum.

Wadeson, H. 1980. *Art psychotherapy.* New York: Wiley.
An overview of contemporary uses of art therapy, for the professional psychotherapist or one interested in training as an art therapist.

Fink, P., and E. Wallace, eds. *The arts in psychotherapy.* (Quarterly journal.) Fayetteville, N.Y.: Ankho International.

Watkins, M. 1976. *Waking dreams.* New York: Harper Colophon Books.

———. 1981. Six approaches to the image in art therapy. *Spring:* 107–25.

Weaver, R. 1977. *The wise old woman: A study of active imagination.* London: Vincent Stuart.
A report of the development and unfolding of a personal myth using active imagination and art materials. The analyst's contribution in tracing mythic parallels links the story to the general human condition.

Wickes, F. 1963. *The inner world of choice.* New York: Harper & Row.

———. 1968. *The inner world of childhood.* New York: Mentor. First ed., 1927, New York: Appleton.

Supplement

On Active Imagination

Marie-Louise von Franz

In this paper (1) I would like to concentrate on what is specific about our active imagination compared to the many other imaginative techniques which are coming to the fore all over the world. We often meet people today who have already practised some such technique before their Jungian analysis and I find it very difficult to teach them how to proceed towards "real" active imagination. I propose therefore to subdivide active imagination into four different stages.

I. First one must empty one's mind from the trains of thought of the ego. This is already very difficult for some people who cannot stop what the Zen-Buddhists aptly call the "mad mind". It is easier to do it in painting and still easier in sand play, but the latter only offers already existing images to the mind so that this first phase of "barrenness" is somewhat omitted, which is apt to lead to difficulties later, when the analysand should proceed to "real" active imagination. Most of the Eastern techniques of meditation, such as Zen, Yoga-practises, Tao-ist meditation, etc., confront us with that first step. In Zen, one is not only taught to stop one's ego-ruminating but also to stop all phantasies which well up from the unconscious. One has either to keep them out by concentrating on a ko'an or to let them flow by and ignore them. The outer "sitting"-exercises are only to be understood as a symbolic expression of this immobilizing of all ego activity.

II. Then comes the second step: It is the phase of letting an unconscious phantasy image enter into the field of inner attention. In contrast to all Eastern techniques we welcome this image and do not dispel or ignore it. We focus on it, and here one has to look out for two kinds of mistake: either one focuses too much and thus arrests the image, fixing it literally so to speak, or one focuses too little and then the inner images are apt to change too quickly—a kind of "inner cinema" begins to run. In my experience, it is especially intuitive types who tend to fall into this trap. They write endless phantastic stories with not much point or rather they do not *relate* to what happens. This

The publisher is grateful for permission to reprint this essay from *Methods of Treatment in Analytical Psychology* (Stuttgart: Verlag Adolf Bonz, 1980), pp. 88–99. The essay originally appeared as "Bemerkungen zur aktiven Imagination," *Analytische Psychologie*, 9 (1978): 161–71, © S. Karger AG (Basel).

is the stage of passive imagination the "imaginatio phantastica" in contrast to the "imaginatio vera". Nowadays this is widely practised in Germany as the "Katathyme Bilderleben" of H. Leuner (2). Leuner took his idea admittedly from Jung and decided to simplify Jung's rather difficult technique, with a very bad result. I find it extremely difficult to teach analysands who have practised this form of imagination. The next step to a real active imagination. W. L. Furrers *Objektivierung des Unbewußten*, Bern 1969 (and Neue *Wege zum Unbewußten*, Bern 1970) stops short at the same point. So does the older technique of Le rêve éveillé de René Desoille. These techniques also allow an interference of the analyst (3)—a great mistake of which I will speak later.

III. Now comes the third step. This consists in giving the phantasy some form of expression: in writing it down, painting it, sculpting or noting the music which one heard, or in dancing it. In the latter case the body comes into it which is sometimes very necessary, mainly when the emotions and the inferior function are so unconscious that they are practically "buried" in the body (4). It often also helps to perform a small ritual like lighting a candle, walking in a circle etc. because through it *matter* enters the play. Jung once told me that this was more efficient than "ordinary active imagination" but he could not explain why.

In my opinion this also answers a problem which is sometimes raised nowadays, the question of the involvement of the body. Actually the alchemistic work is nothing else than an active imagination according to Jung performed by the mixing, heating etc. of material substances. The Eastern alchemists, mainly Taoistic, usually did this by trying to influence the matter of their own body, but also that of the materials in their retorts. The Western alchemists mostly used matter outside their body, asserting that "our soul imagines great things outside the body" (extra corpus). Paracelsus and his pupil Gerhard Dorn however also tried to experiment with "the inner firmament" within their own bodies with some outer magical performances; these had—per analogy—a synchronistic relationship to the matter in the body. Thus active imagination is actually very much concerned with the body but essentially with its basic chemical components in their symbolic meaning. I have often observed strong physical positive and negative reactions in case of a rightly or wrongly conducted active imagination; one analysand even once suffered a severe but purely psychogenic heart-attack, when he betrayed his feelings within an active imagination (5). A great problem is raised by strong affects and emotions. In his own experiment Jung sometimes used yoga exercises to master them first, before he could, so to speak, extract an image from them to which he could relate in active imagination (6). Certain active imaginations can be done as conversations with inwardly perceived parts of one's body, or hearing them speak. This can be especially helpful in cases of a psychogenic physical symptom. Whenever matter is touched upon, be it inside or outside one's own body, there is a chance that markedly numerous synchronistic events will occur, which shows that this form of active imagination is especially powerful. On the negative side it touches upon the subject of magic and its dangers to which I will return later.

On this level two major mistakes can occur as Jung points out in his paper on the "Transcendent Function" (7): either one gives the phantasy too much aesthetical elaboration, it becomes a "piece of art" and in one's eagerness to cope with the form one overlooks the message or meaning of it. This happens in my experience mostly with painting and writing. Too much form kills the content just as art has in many historical periods "buried the gods in gold and marble," so that one prefers to see a primitive fetish or the clumsy art of the early Christians. Sensations and feeling mainly lead us astray in this respect. One forgets that what one creates is only a replica of an inner reality and that the aim is to relate to the latter, not the replica. The other mistake is the reverse: one sketches the phantasy-content only in a sloppy way and jumps at once to asking after its meaning. This is a danger which mostly threatens intuitive and thinking types and worst: the intellectuals. It shows a lack of love and devotion. One can see it at once when a patient brings a sloppy sketch or a badly written bit of paper with an air of knowing already what it means. This third step which lends the unconscious a mode of self-expression in creative form brings generally already a great release. However, it is not yet "real" active imagination.

IV. The fourth step is the decisive one, the step where most other modern parallel techniques miss out. It is the *ethical confrontation* with whatever one has previously produced. Here Jung warns against a most frequent and fatal mistake: namely that one enters the "inner play" with a fictitious ego and not with one's own true ego (8).

Let me give an example: an analysand dreamt that he found in a desert a horse's hoof, which was highly dangerous. It began to pursue him. It was a sort of Wotanic demon. In active imagination he continued the dream. He ran away on a horse. The horse foot-demon began to become bigger and bigger and came always closer. Then the patient turned and somehow overcame it and stamped it into the ground. When the analysand told me this story, I felt a strange discrepancy between his actual looks and the outcome of the story. He looked deeply worried and anxious. I told him that I did not believe that it happened as in the story but I could not tell why. A week later he confessed that when the horse foot-demon reached him, he became split: only one part of him overcame the demon, the other part "jumped out of the drama" and was only looking on at the scene. So the victory over the demon had been only achieved by a fictitious heroic ego, his real ego just jumped out and secretly thought: "This is only a phantasy." In my experience—when the actual observable emotional state of the analysand's ego does not coincide with that in the story one can see that the drama was only lived through by a fictitious ego. This mistake is very difficult to detect. Another analysand had a long love affair with an anima figure in an active imagination. But he never told her that he was married. When I asked him he said he would never do this in reality. So his ego in the active imagination behaved differently to his every day-ego. The whole thing was obviously not quite real, it was more like writing a novel, but not an actual active imagination. This is most important because the effectiveness of active imagination depends entirely on this point. Very split people and people threatened by a latent psychosis generally cannot do active imagination at all or they do it in this fictitious way and nothing comes of it. As you know Jung warned against letting borderline cases do active imagination altogether. The second example which I gave does not concern a sick analysand but an intellectual. The intellect is a great trickster who can make one quite inadvertently overlook the moral issue and sneaks the semi-unconscious thought into one's head that it is all "phantasy" or "wishful thinking" and thus undoes the whole thing. It needs a certain naiveté to do real active imagination.

Jung once remarked that in psychiatry nowadays, one has generally discovered the proceeding up to the third step but that the fourth is not understood. All the techniques which I mentioned before stop short before this fourth step. Another point that is not yet realized is that in most of the before-mentioned therapeutical creative-phantasy-techniques a certain interference of the analyst is permitted or even called for. Either the analyst suggests a theme as in Carl Happich's technique (9) or in the advanced stages of J. H. Schultz's "autogenic training," or he intervenes when the analysand gets stuck and suggests an issue. Jung on the contrary left the patient stuck, right up against the wall, until he found an issue for himself. He told us once how he had a patient who in life always fell into the same trap. He told her to do an active imagination. She promptly had the phantasy that she came in a field up to a high wall and knew that she should get to the other side, but she did not know how. Jung only said: "What would you do in reality?" She could not think of anything. He left her there. Finally she thought of walking along and looking if the wall ended somewhere. It did not. Then she looked for a door or window. There was none. Again she was stuck for a very long time, but Jung did not help. Finally she thought of fetching a hammer and chisel and making a hole into the wall; this worked and she could get on. The fact that the woman could not imagine such a simple thing mirrors the inner fact that she behaved exactly in the same way in outer reality. It is therefore essential *not to interfere with a helpful suggestion,* which would keep her just as helpless, infantile and passive as before. On the contrary if she learnt the hard way within the active imagination to overcome the obstacle, she would have also learnt something for outer life. Even if a patient was stuck in active imagination over weeks Jung did not give a helpful suggestion but insisted that he or she should continue to struggle with the problem himself and alone.

In controlled drug-taking this fourth step is again missed. The controlling person carries the responsibility instead of the producer of the phantasy. I came across an interesting book by two brothers Terence and Denis McKenna: *The Invisible Landscape* (10). These two courageous young men went to Mexico and experimented on themselves with a hallucinogenic plant. They experienced according to their own report schizophrenic states of mind, which led to a great widening of consciousness. Unfortunately they could not keep track of the experiences except that they went to other planets and were often helped by an invisible guide who was sometimes a huge insect. The second part of the book contains the speculations which they derived from their visions. *They are not different from any other wildly intuitive modern speculations about mind, matter, synchronicity etc.* In other words they do not actually convey anything really new or which the two well-read authors could not have thought out consciously. But what is decisive is the fact that the book ends with the idea that all life on earth will be definitely destroyed in an approaching cataclysm and that we must either find means to escape to another planet or turn inward and escape into the realm of the cosmic mind. Let me compare this with a dream which an American student allowed me to use and which is concerned with the same theme. This student, let me remark, is in no way psychotic and is in a Jungian analysis. He dreamt:

I am walking along what appears to be the Palisades, overlooking all of New York City. I am walking with an anima figure who is unknown to me personally; we are both being led by a man who is our guide. NYC is in a rubble—the world in fact has been destroyed as we know it. All of NYC is just one heap of wreckage, there are fires everywhere, thousands of people are running in every direction frantically, the Hudson river has over-flowed many areas of the city, smoke is billowing up everywhere. As far as I can see the land has been leveled. It was twilight; fireballs were in the sky, heading for the earth. It was the end of the world, total destruction of everything that man and his civilization had built up.

The cause of this great destruction was a race of great giants—giants who had come from outer space—from the far reaches of the universe. In the middle of the rubble I could see two of them sitting; they were casually scooping up people by the handful and eating them. All this was done with the same nonchalance that we have when we sit down at the table and eat grapes by the handful. The sight was awesome. The giants were not the same size or quite the same structure. Our guide explained that the giants were from different planets and live harmoniously and peacefully together. The guide also explained that the giants landed in flying saucers (the fireballs were other landings). In fact the earth as we know it was conceived by this race of giants in the beginning of time as we know it. They cultivated our civilization, like we cultivate vegetables in a hot house. The earth was their hot house, so-to-speak, and now they have returned to reap the fruits they have sown, but there was a special occasion for all this which I wasn't to become aware of till later.

I was saved because I had slightly high blood pressure. If I had normal blood pressure or if my blood pressure was too high I would have been eaten like almost all the others. But because I have slightly high blood pressure (hypertension) I am chosen to go through this ordeal, and if I pass the ordeal I would become like my guide, "a saver of souls". We walked for an extraordinarily long time, witnessing all the cataclysmic destruction. Then before me I saw a huge golden throne, it was as brilliant as the sun, impossible to view straight on. On the throne sat a King and his Queen of the race of giants. They were the intelligence behind the destruction of our planet as I know it. There was something special or extraordinary about them which I didn't become aware of till later.

The ordeal, in addition to witnessing the world's destruction, or task I had to perform was to climb up this staircase until I was at their level—"face to face" with them. This was probably in stages. I started climbing, it was long and very difficult, my heart was pounding very hard. I felt frightened but knew I had to accomplish this task, the world and humanity was at stake. I woke up from this dream perspiring heavily.

Later I realized that the destruction of the earth by the race of giants was a wedding feast for the newly united King and Queen, this was the special occasion and the extraordinary feeling I had about the King and Queen.

The giants had elongated heads, with humanoid bodies. The back of their heads were elongated and the lower front part was extended. They had no eyes in their sockets, but had a piece of skin where eyes are, through which they had vision as we normally know it, in addition to some special kind of perception process that could project images telepathically into others' image receivers. There was no external ear structure, although there was an internal ear, also no nostrils were protruding and yet there was some kind of internal nose structure. The skin looked taut and in plate-like segments, four sides to each segment that narrowed towards the front of the face. The mouth seemed similar to ours. I don't remember any hair; some kind of one piece suit was worn which looked like a combination of rubber and silicon; it seemed to be unaffected by fire, water, or anything that hit it. (End of dream).

This scene reminds one of the invasion of giants in the book of Enoch, which Jung interpreted as a "premature invasion of the collective unconscious," which caused a general inflation. The angels who generated the giants with mortal women also taught men a lot of scientific knowledge which caused their inflation. It is clear that this dream mirrors our similar modern situation and the book of the McKennas' among others shows clearly how such premature exploiting of visions of the collective unconscious leads into dangerous states of mind.

The great difference between this dream and the drug phantasies of the McKenna brothers lies in the fact that there is a *task* set for the dreamer, namely to reach the King and Queen who are on earth for their wedding. In the McKennas' phantasies there is nothing to be done for the individual, he can only run away, if possible, or succumb. A more constructive aspect of the unconscious is probably only constellated when it has a conscious ego as vis-à-vis. The same holds true for active imagination and this is why controlled drug-taking as well as active imagination in which the analyst participates are not the right thing. The ego remains infantile and will fall into the same traps as it did before, as soon as it is left to itself again.

The apocalyptic view of an end of the world in *The Invisible Landscape* and in our dream are related to all our apprehensions about a third world war. But the difference is striking: instead of an escape into outer space or into the spiritual realm, the dreamer is burdened with the heavy task of reaching the King and Queen. They represent the uniting of the opposites, of Father and Mother, Spirit and Matter. This reminds me that Jung once said, when we asked him about another war to come, that in his opinion another war could only be avoided if enough individuals were standing the tension and holding the opposites together in themselves. The whole task is now put on the shoulders of the individual and one can understand the fears of our dreamer. But the unconscious can only sketch a way out for us *if we are and remain individually conscious.*

One important motif of the dream is the guide who turns up and leads the dreamer. This can only happen when the analyst does not push himself in as a guide. That is why one should not interfere in active imagination; not even a little bit! Hermes, the guide of the alchemists, said that he was "the friend of anybody who was alone" (cuius que segregati—of everyone who is separated from the flock!). One essential effect of active imagination is, according to Jung, that it enables the analysand to become independent of the analyst—so if one interferes, everything is spoilt. (This naturally does not mean that one must not interfere when the analysand does some wrong kind of imagination). When an analysand reads an active imagination he has had to me, I often think silently at certain points: "Oh I would not have done (or said) that." This shows one how individual the ego's reaction to the inner figures is and that this reaction should come completely and only from the analysand is therefore essential. It decides the "turns" which the course of the active imagination takes.

An interesting new (or rather age old) attempt towards active imagination is described in Carlos Castaneda's tales about Don Juan's, the Indian sorcerer, method of what he calls "Dreaming". This seems to be based on older Mexican medicine mens' traditions. It is as you know now very much read by the younger generation in America. "Dreaming" is an active imagination which is performed with phenomena, which one encounters in nature. The Indian master Don Juan takes Castaneda for a walk in the completely deserted wild chaparral in the dusk. Suddenly Castaneda sees a dark shape of what he thinks is a dying animal. He gets terrified and wants to run away, but then he looks once more a bit more closely and discovers that it is only a dead branch. Don Juan says afterwards (11): "What you have done is no triumph. You've wasted a beautiful power that blew life into that dry twig . . . That branch was a real animal and it was alive at the moment the power touched it. Since what kept it alive was power, the trick was, like in dreaming, to sustain the sight of it."

What Don Juan calls power is mana, mulungu, in other words the active energy-aspect of the unconscious. By rationalizing his fearful phantasy, Castaneda has chased away this power so he lost his chance to learn how "to stop the world". (This is Don Juan's expression for stopping the ego's train of thought). Don Juan calls this form of "Dreaming" also "controlled folly" which reminds one of Jung calling active imagination a "voluntary psychosis". This doing the active imagination with outer phenomena in nature reminds one of the alchemists who operated with metal, plants and stones, but the difference is that the alchemists always had a *vessel*. This vessel is the "imaginatio vera" or the "theoria," they did not get lost, but had a "comprehension" in the literal sense of the word, a religious philosophy. Don Juan has one too, but he cannot convey it to Castaneda and thus remains the controlling guide.

As I mentioned before, this ritual form of active imagination is especially powerful but also dangerous. It constellates a lot of synchronistic events, which can easily be misunderstood as magic. And psychotic people tend to misinterpret them most dangerously. I remember the case of a man, who in the beginning of an episode attacked his wife. She called for the police and a psychiatrist. When the two arrived and they were all standing in the passage of the flat, the only electric light bulb exploded and they were all plunged in darkness and splinters. The man interpreted it in this way: He was the saviour and just as Sun and Moon were eclipsed when Christ was crucified, so now darkness came when he was unjustly arrested. However the synchronistic event contained on the contrary a healthy message, it warned him that the light of his ego consciousness was exploding—just what it did and he fell into a mental blackout. You see how much one moves here on dangerous ground. Though this incident did not happen in an active imagination but in a state near psychosis, it is apt to illuminate what kind of error can happen in the state of "voluntary psychosis," the excitement over synchronistic happenings blurs one's judgement of what it could mean. That is why Zosimos warns against demons which can interfere with the alchemical opus. Here we touch upon nothing less than the difference between magic especially black magic and active imagination. As you know Jung advised his pupils against doing active imagination with living persons. This is because it can have magical effects upon them and also because magic, even "white magic," *has often a boomerang-effect on the one who exercises it*. It is therefore destructive to oneself in the long run. I remember however one incident where Jung advised me to do it: I had an analysand who was so totally animus possessed that she was no longer accessible and was close to drowning in a psychotic state. Jung advised me to do an active imagination with her animus. It would help, but it would do *me* harm. However it was a last resort, so I should do it only as an exception. It had in fact a salutary effect upon the analysand and Jung then helped me out of the boomerang-effect, but I never dared to do it again. The borderline between active imagination and magic is sometimes very subtle. In magic there is always a *desire* or *wish* of the ego involved, either a "good intention" or an evil destructive wish. I have also seen that strong animus or anima possession generally prevents people from being able to do active imagination. Both destroy the objectivity of the ego which is needed. One should do the latter with the object of getting near the truth and only the truth about oneself. But in practice some desirousness often sneaks in from behind and then one falls into the "imaginatio phantastica" instead of "imaginatio vera". I have noticed a similar danger in casting the I Ching. If one is in a mood of desirousness one misinterprets its oracles. The reverse danger is that one doubts too much what one hears or sees in active imagination, thinking that it is only wishful phantasizing. Generally this is cured by some turn in the active imagination which comes as such a surprise that one gets convinced of not having made it up.

Finally, there is one more step about active imagination namely that one has to apply whatever is said, ordered or asked for in active imagination to ordinary life. I remember a case of a man who promised his anima in an active imagination to speak at least ten minutes with her every day in the immediate future. He then neglected it and fell into a very neurotic state before he realized that it had been caused by his having broken his promise. But this is naturally true for all realizations in analysis.

This is so to speak the opening of the retort in alchemy; something which just naturally follows if one has really understood the former steps. If people don't do it, then they actually have not achieved the fourth step of a real ethical confrontation.

REFERENCES

(1) First published in the "Analytische Psychologie," ed. Biller, Dieckmann & Meier. S. Karger AG, Basel 1978.

(2) H. Leuner, *Katathymes Bilderleben*. Unterstufe. Ein Seminar-Kurs. Thieme, Stuttgart 1970.

(3) Cf. for instance Ilse Henle, "Die Anwendung des Katathymen Bilderlebens bei der Therapie ehelicher Virginität" in *Materialien zur Psychoanalyse und analytisch orientierten Psychotherapie*, ed. Hahn-Herdieckerhoff. Vaudenhoeck, Göttingen-Zürich 1977, III. Serie. 4. Lieferung.

(4) Cf. also Elie G. Humbert, L'imagination active d'après C. G. Jung. Cahiers de Psychologie Jungienne. Paris. and the literature stated here.

(5) See M.-L. von Franz, "Active Imagination in der Psychologie von C. G. Jung" in: *Geist und Psyche*, ed. Bitter. Kindler Taschenbücher (without date).

(6) See *Memories, Dreams, Reflections*, ed. A. Jaffé. Passim.

(7) Collected Works, Vol. 8 (1916–1957). In "Spring 1971" R. F. C. Hull has assembled a bibliography of all texts of Jung on active imagination (p. 115 ff.).

(8) *Mysterium Coniunctionis*, Collected Works Vol. 14, last 3 chapters.

(9) Cf. W. Kretschmer, "Die meditativen Verfahren in der Psychotherapie". Zeitschrift für Psychotherapie und medizinische Psychologie. Bd. I, No. 3, Mai, 1951.

(10) Seabury Press, New York 1975.

(11) Carlos Castaneda, *Journey to Ixtlan*, Simon and Schuster, New York 1972, pp. 132–3.